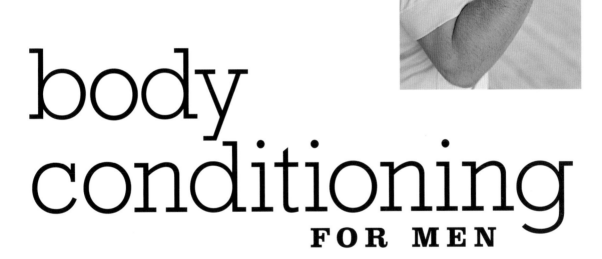

body
conditioning
FOR MEN

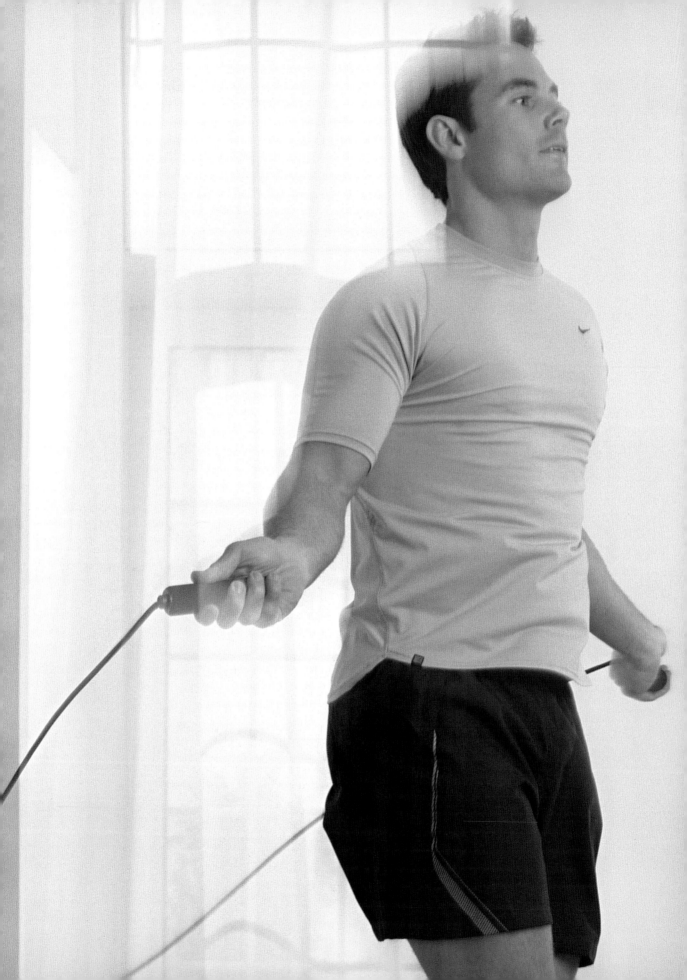

body conditioning

FOR MEN

Get fit and **stay fit** using the progressive 12–week programme

Paul Stephen Lubicz

hamlyn

I would like to dedicate this book to Ernest Graham, who believed that exercise had no age barriers!

First published in Great Britain in 2005 by
Hamlyn, a division of Octopus Publishing Group Limited
2–4 Heron Quays, London E14 4JP

ISBN 0 600 61005 5
EAN 9780600610052

A CIP catalogue record for this book is available from the British Library

Printed and bound in China

10 9 8 7 6 5 4 3 2 1

Note

It is advisable to check with your doctor before embarking on any exercise programme. A physician should be consulted on all matters relating to health and any symptoms which may require diagnosis or medical attention. While the advice and information in this book is believed to be accurate and the instructions given have been devised to avoid strain, neither the author nor the publisher can accept any legal responsibility for any injury sustained while following the exercises.

contents

introduction

We have all heard the conventional wisdom for building a fit and healthy body – undertake 30 minutes of cardiovascular exercise five times a week, do weight training to build and tone muscle, drink water, avoid alcohol and eat sensibly. Motivating yourself to undergo such a lifestyle overhaul at the same time as managing job, family and other commitments can be very daunting and seem too big a prospect to handle.

In addition, the often contradictory and ever changing suggestions put forward by the media for diet and exercise regimes can be confusing and unrealistic for most people. To make matters worse, the exaggerated importance given to body appearance often eclipses the importance of life balance, physical health and peace of mind.

The aim of my body conditioning programme is to enable you to balance the responsibilities and demands of your daily life with a consistent approach to exercise and healthy lifestyle choices, which will result in an improved quality of life. I have designed the programme to be easy to understand, fun and motivating. It delivers a fantastic workout, allowing those of you not used to exercising to progress from the beginner level, through to the intermediate level and on to a more advanced exercise platform.

Move more

My body conditioning programme is a progressive training plan that will improve your general condition and wellbeing as you make advances in your training. However, I also really want to emphasize the advantages of being more active in your everyday life. The opportunities are limitlessness, so make it a daily challenge to find ways to move your body.

You don't have to join a health club or attend an aerobics class and you don't have to wear special clothes or perform complicated activities. It can be as simple as choosing between parking right next to your destination or parking farther away and walking a little, choosing between sleeping in at the weekend or washing the car, or taking the stairs whenever there is a choice between stairs and escalators or elevators. Walk wherever and whenever you can – walk your dog, mow the lawn, kick a football with friends and chase your kids. When was the last time you played tag around the park? Give it a go – you will be amazed at what a great workout it is!

Remember that any activity that moves your limbs is not only a fitness tool, it can also be a stress buster. In addition, you can think 'move' in small increments of time. It doesn't have to be an hour in the gym or a 45-minute kickboxing class. These are great forms of exercise but realistically not always possible to fit in your day. Simply move more and take every opportunity to burn calories and improve your general fitness and you will feel better.

Everyone can do it

Exercise is often associated with young people, but there is no reason why it cannot be enjoyed by all ages. However old you are, you can improve your strength, endurance and flexibility by becoming more active. A carefully chosen exercise regime can have a large impact on someone in their later years, with the result that they feel better and get around more easily.

People with physical limitations and chronic conditions can also benefit by becoming more active. Increasing your level of physical activity as much as you are able can help to offset many of the negative effects of certain diseases and disabling conditions. By getting out to exercise, you'll meet new people, have fun, feel more relaxed and sleep better.

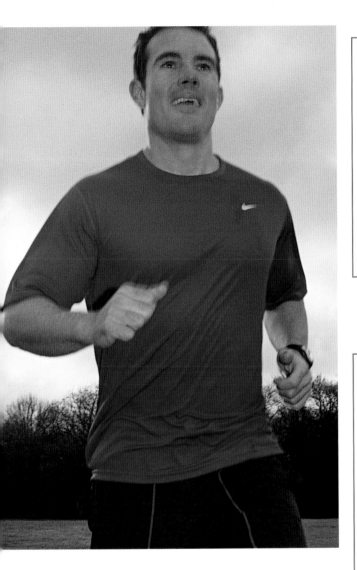

Every day you have the option of being more active, and everyone can benefit from increased physical activity.

benefits of increased mobility

- Better physical and mental health
- Improved quality of life and self-esteem
- Increased energy
- Reduced stress
- Better posture and balance
- Stronger muscles and bones; fewer aches and pains
- Good weight maintenance
- More active older adults have the function and fitness of much younger people
- Prolonged independent living

safety precautions

Before starting any new training or lifestyle programme I strongly recommend that you seek approval from your medical practitioner. This will give you peace of mind and allow you to receive any relevant medical information that could affect your ability to exercise. It is also a good idea to get a postural assessment (see page 27) from a qualified movement screening professional or exercise specialist before starting an exercise programme, so that any muscular imbalances may be detected and corrected before an injury occurs. You definitely need a check-up from your doctor before exercising if you:

- Have been diagnosed with heart problems, high blood pressure, diabetes or any other serious medical condition or illness
- Experience chest pain, dizziness or fainting spells
- Are recovering from an injury or illness
- Are over 65 and do not currently exercise
- Have been sedentary for over a year

motivating yourself

Setting yourself appropriate goals will give you the motivation to start your exercise programme. Achieving challenging, realistic short-term goals along the way will help keep you motivated, giving you the incentive and drive to continue your programme and to work towards more long-term goals such as improved quality of life.

Planning to be successful is the key.
Setting short-term goals, even on a daily basis, will help map out a path to reach your full potential.

Setting yourself goals

I am a strong believer in goal setting. I believe that if we don't know what we want or where we want to go, the chances are that we will not get anywhere. The process of setting a goal requires us to crystallize and conceptualize what we may want subconsciously into something we are actively willing to seek on a conscious level. For the goal to last, it must emerge from some deep-felt desire. If you get in touch with what you really want, setting a coinciding goal will follow naturally.

It is not only important to set goals, it is imperative that they are realistic. However, there must be a balance. Accomplishing a goal that is not challenging is not fulfilling. Conversely, setting a goal that is too challenging is a set-up for failure.

Take time to think about your desire to get fit – what does 'get fit' really mean to you? Do you mean that you would like to tone up? Would like to be able to run a marathon? To achieve success in anything you need to have a plan; then, once your direction is clear, the trip will be that much easier to maintain and follow.

So, set yourself a realistic goal that is challenging and stick to your training and eating programme. Regularly step out of your comfort zone and push for higher achievement. Aim for consistency rather than perfection. Being perfect is not a realistic goal, so setting such a high standard for yourself could actually reverse your progress. It is consistency of exercise that achieves results.

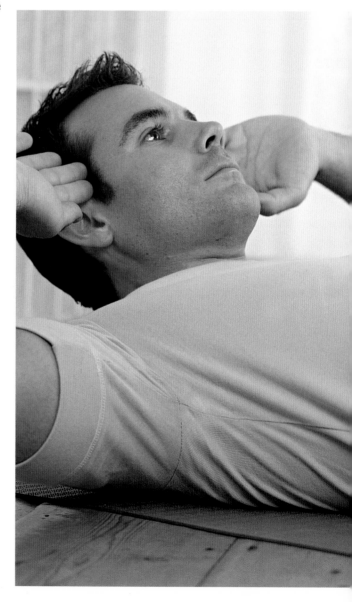

How to achieve your goal

Achieving your desired goal will come down to keeping a positive mental attitude and breaking down your goal into short-term targets on a daily basis. Combine consistent, passionate action with clear direction and positive self-belief, and you will create a recipe for success in whatever you do. Visualize yourself accomplishing your goal and pick a goal that you can

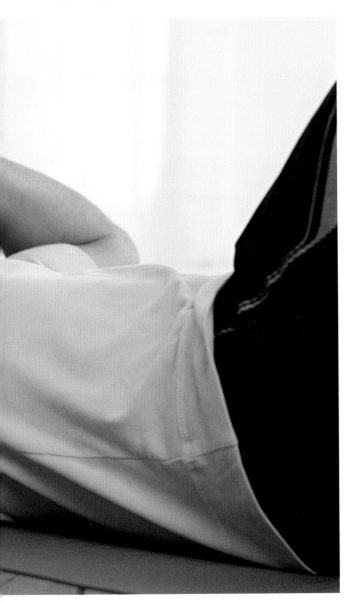

measure and gauge your progress towards. Even if your overall goal is not definitive, it is helpful to create milestones and mini victories for yourself that will build momentum towards your ultimate goal. Don't forget to enjoy the feeling of mastering these challenges. Let that build your confidence to tackle your next hurdle. Having confidence will give you the power to take on the goals you set yourself.

In addition, find an emotional reason to keep on target, something that will make a difference in your life. Your emotions are a very powerful force and will help you in your drive towards success. It also helps to have a great support team – lean on friends and family and gain inspiration and strength from their stability.

Bear in mind that boredom can destroy your enthusiasm – same routine, same results. Try something different and you will get different results, so make sure that you enjoy your exercise programme!

tips for successful training

- Buy a small notebook to keep track of your workouts, to help you be more consistent
- Find a workout buddy to keep you motivated
- Get professional advice from a personal trainer or nutritionist. Starting out on the right foot can make exercise more effective and more fun
- Be consistent. Stick with it and you'll see results
- Be more active generally in everyday life. The more you get your body moving, the more energy you'll have to fulfil your daily obligations. Exercise also helps you sleep better and it keeps you alert all day long
- Aim for consistency not perfection

anatomy

The human body is made up of a
number of complex body systems, all
of which work together to make us
function efficiently and healthily. To
help you understand just some of
the body's amazing anatomy, the
major muscles referred to throughout
the book are described below.

Triceps
Location The back of the upper arms.
Motion performed The triceps
straighten your arms when you push
yourself off the floor when performing
a press-up.

Rhomboids
Location Two muscles in the centre of
the upper back.
Motion performed The rhomboids
help control and stabilize your shoulder
blades (the wing-shaped bones behind
the shoulders).

Buttock muscles, or glutes (gluteals)
Location The bottom.
Motion performed The gluteals assist
in extension of the hip, for example
when you rise out of a seat, and are used
when you move your leg behind you.

Hamstrings
Location The back of the thighs.
Motion performed The hamstrings
bend the knees and help decelerate the
body when squatting.

Inner thigh muscles
Location The groin.
Motion performed The inner thigh
(groin) muscles bring your legs in
towards your body.

Calf muscles
Location The back of the lower leg.
Motion performed The calves allow
you to reach high on your toes to reach a
top shelf and also stabilize your ankles
when you walk.

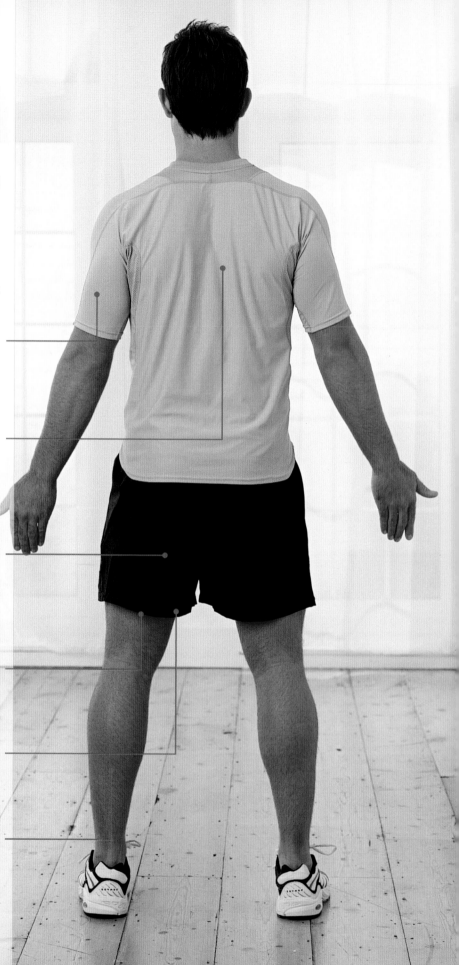

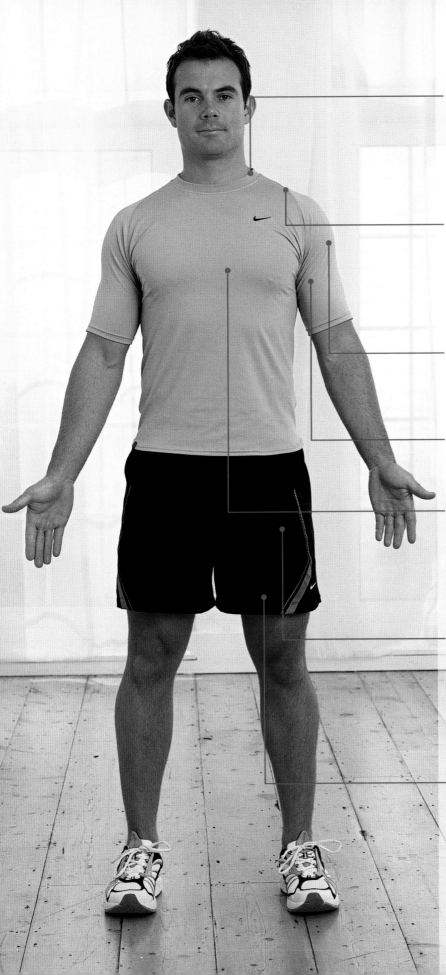

Levator scapulae

Location The small muscles that run up either side of your neck from the top of the shoulder blades to just below your ears.

Motion performed The levator scapulae are used when you move your head bilaterally.

Trapezius muscles

Location The large muscles that run from either side of the back of the neck towards your shoulders and down into the middle of the back.

Motion performed You use the trapezius muscles when you shrug your shoulders.

Shoulder muscles

Location At the very top of the arms.

Motion performed The shoulder muscles move your upper arms up, back and to the side.

Biceps

Location The front of the upper arms.

Motion performed The biceps allow you to bend your arms into your body.

Chest muscles, or pecs (pectorals)

Location The upper chest, in line with the heart.

Motion performed When all the fibres work together, the pecs bring your arms across your body. You use them to throw a basketball or push a lawn mower.

Hips, or hip flexors

Location The front of the hips. To locate your hip flexors, place your hands beneath the front part of your hip bone at the top front of the leg.

Motion performed The hip flexors help decelerate your hips when you sit down and help you to lift your knees up to your chest.

Front thigh muscles, or quads (quadriceps)

Location The muscles on the front of the thighs.

Motion performed The quads straighten your legs and you use them every time you take a step.

essential equipment

The following items of fitness equipment are all light or compact and portable, and can be used to provide a great workout at home, in the office or in the park – proving that exercise can be done virtually anywhere.

Swiss ball

The Swiss ball, also known as an exercise ball or a stability ball, is an effective tool for fitness training. Physiotherapists have used them for years, but fitness experts now recognize that a Swiss ball is one of the best ways to strengthen the body's core and increase stability while looking after posture.

A Swiss ball is a good substitute for gym equipment in your home. You can buy Swiss balls at most department or fitness stores, at some gyms and via the internet. Check that the ball is durable and can support your body weight and additional loads if you will be using free weights. Also make sure that it is the right size for your height. To test it, sit on the ball and ensure your knees are bent at about 90°. The following chart will help you find the perfect fit:

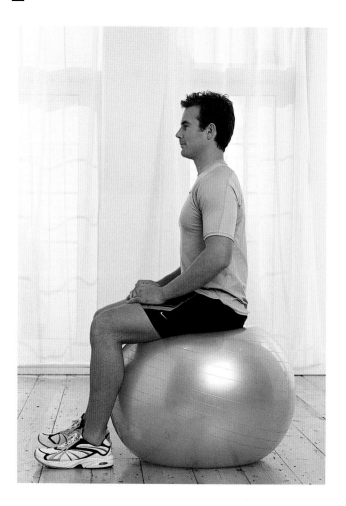

Ball size	User height
55 cm (22 in)	1.50–1.64 m (4 ft 11 in–5 ft 4 in)
65 cm (26 in)	1.65–1.81 m (5 ft 5 in–5 ft 11 in)
75 cm (30 in)	1.82–2.00 m (6 ft 0 in–6 ft 7 in)

Resistance band

The great thing about the rubber resistance band is that it offers a progressive resistance level for multiple users and fitness levels. It allows the isolation of targeted muscle groups and works well with a full range of motion exercises. The band is versatile and travels well – it can be folded up and fitted into a small bag. All you need is a little space to use it for a safe and effective body conditioning workout.

A Swiss ball is one of the best ways to strengthen the body's core and increase stability while looking after posture.

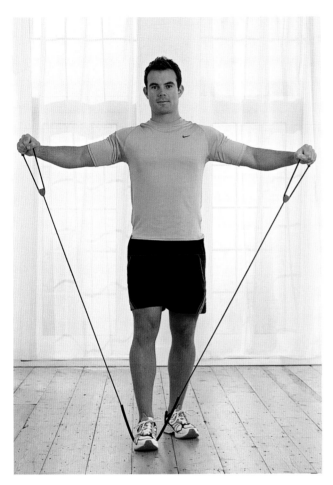

away when placed on the floor. Dumbbells with an adjustable weight stack are another option, for example the PowerBlock dumbbell with its selector pin system. The versatility of such dumbbells makes them great for home use because they require less storage space than a set of dumbbells of different weights and can be used by the whole family.

Dumbbells are also very compatible with various other pieces of fitness equipment, for example with a bench for strength training and with a Swiss ball for stability and balance development.

Foam rolls

Foam rolls are 15 cm (6 in) in diameter and come in two different lengths: 30 cm (1 ft) and 90 cm (3 ft) long. They are used for self-myofascial release (self-massage) (see pages 28–29 and 44–53), and can also be used for balance training and for improving posture and alignment. The smaller size is ideal if you will be travelling with your foam roll.

Exercise mat

Mats are ideal for keeping you clean and comfortable while you are stretching or doing floor exercises. Choose a mat made of closed cell foam, which is easy to wipe clean and won't absorb moisture, and that is guaranteed for a decent length of time and thick enough not to be easily torn and damaged. Also bear in mind the size of your mat – one that is 5 cm (2 in) thick and 1.2 m (4 ft) long will roll up, transport and store well.

Dumbbells

An excellent form of resistance training, dumbbell exercises create instability, forcing the body to balance and strengthen itself through multiple planes of motion.

Dumbbell training is effective and safe for all applications and users – the weights available cater for beginners through to strength athletes.

The equipment is easily available and the cost is low. There are different dumbbells to choose from – plated loaded dumbbells (these have a collar, which secures weights to a small dumbbell bar) and solid 'hex' dumbbells being the most common. The hexagonal shape of the latter prevents the dumbbells from rolling

nutrition

Good nutrition is a vital part of health and fitness. Healthy eating can help you lose, maintain or gain weight in the right way, reduce your risk of diseases such as heart disease, diabetes and cancer and support the demands of exercise and training. Healthy eating can give you more energy, put you in a better mood and help you feel great!

What is a healthy diet?

A healthy balanced diet provides all the nutrients you need and is best achieved by eating a wide variety of foods. The principal components of foods are proteins, fats and carbohydrates. These 'macronutrients' provide energy, which is measured in calories. Fat is the most energy-dense nutrient and provides 9 calories per gram, whereas protein and carbohydrate provide 4 calories per gram. Food also contains vitamins and minerals, classed as 'micronutrients', which are needed in only small quantities. They do not provide energy, but are essential for the many biochemical processes in the body.

There are no guarantees in life and your genetics have a great influence on your longevity but you can help yourself by watching what you eat. Not only are you likely to improve your health, but good nutrition will also support your training diet and help condition your body.

good eating habits

- Cut excess visible fat from meat, e.g. steak and bacon
- Choose grilled food more often than fried
- Include vegetables or a salad with every meal
- Select fruit as a snack and to follow meals
- Eat oil-rich fish, e.g. salmon, pilchards, mackerel or sardines, twice a week
- Drink plenty of water
- Ensure you have some alcohol-free days

The heart of the matter

A healthy diet can help you reduce three of the major risk factors for a heart attack – high blood pressure, high blood cholesterol and too much body fat. Healthy eating need not be complicated and it certainly does not mean that you have to give up any of the foods you like. It is not about banning foods, it just means that some foods should be eaten in larger quantities and more often than others. Simply base your diet on nutrient-dense foods such as fruit and vegetables, oats, wholemeal and wholegrain bread and cereals, low-fat dairy products, fish, lean meats, skinless chicken and beans and pulses. Watch the amount of fat within your diet and try to keep your intake of foods that are high in saturated fats to a minimum. These include full-fat cheeses, fatty meats, butter and butter-like spreads, cakes and biscuits, snack foods like crisps, coconut and vegetable oils not labelled as unsaturated.

Eat a few nuts (high in fibre, vitamin E, potassium and magnesium) several times a week as they can reduce the risk of heart disease. Although nuts are high in fat, it is mainly unsaturated, which may help to reduce cholesterol levels. In addition, moderate the amount of alcohol you drink and try to limit the amount of salt you eat. Garlic has been suggested as a food to lower blood pressure and blood lipids; however, more research is needed to determine the specific effects on blood cholesterol.

Organic food

Your body is a reflection of the quality of the food you eat, so good food is essential. Organic food is grown at a normal rate, which means that the food has time to develop the correct levels of vitamins and minerals. In addition, eating organic produce means that you avoid exposure to a multitude of chemicals.

eat plenty of fruit and vegetables

Eating more fruit and vegetables will help you maintain a healthy weight and may help protect against heart disease and cancer. Fruit and vegetables have plenty of plus points. They are high in fibre, rich in the antioxidant vitamins (vitamins A, C and E) and folate (a B vitamin), most are virtually fat free and low in calories. The following fruit and vegetables are particularly good for us.

Avocados The avocado is one of the few fruits that contains fat but it is the type of fat that keeps you healthy. Avocados contain fibre and vitamin B6 and are a great source of vitamin E, which prolongs the life of red blood cells and helps prevent damage to the cells of the body.

Bananas Bananas are popular with athletes because they are a mix of different types of carbohydrate, which provide sustained energy. A good source of dietary fibre, vitamin C and B6, an average banana provides about 100 calories. They are also a rich source of potassium, which helps keep the heart, nervous system and kidneys healthy.

Broccoli A great source of vitamin C and fibre, and providing iron, potassium, vitamin E, folate and betacarotene, broccoli is low in fat and 100 g (3½ oz) provides just 25 calories. The deeper the colour of the vegetable, the higher its betacarotene content.

Carrots Carrots are an excellent source of betacarotene, which is converted in the body to vitamin A, which helps with night vision. Our bodies absorb more betacarotene from cooked carrots than they do from raw ones.

Green peppers One raw medium sweet green pepper contains 20 calories and is an excellent source of vitamin C and folic acid.

Oranges Just one 180 g (6¾ oz) orange contains 76 mg of vitamin C and 50 calories. Oranges are a good source of fibre and provide some betacarotene, as well as other carotenoids. Their pith and peel are rich in pectin (a type of soluble fibre) and flavonoids, which may be at least partly responsible for the reputation of oranges as being good at preventing colds.

Tomatoes Tomatoes are a rich source of lycopene, a carotenoid that seems to reduce the risk of prostate cancer. The riper the tomato, the higher the level of lycopene. A good source of vitamin C, tomatoes also provide respectable amounts of vitamin E, folate, betacarotene and dietary fibre. Tomatoes are fat free and 100 g (3½ oz) provides 13 calories.

Spring onions Spring onions provide small amounts of many vitamins and minerals and some dietary fibre. They are an excellent source of vitamin C and their green tops contain betacarotene. They are fat free and low in calories, typically providing 27 calories per 100 g (3½ oz).

Eating and exercising

Active men should always eat adequate amounts of carbohydrate to support training and recovery. The amount you need to eat depends upon how often, how hard and how long you train and the type of exercise you are doing.

You should always eat breakfast and have regular meals and snacks throughout the day. Choose plenty of foods high in carbohydrate, for example fruit, bread, rice, pasta, cereals, potatoes, low-fat milk and milkshakes, beans and pulses. Include moderate amounts of food containing protein, for example fish, meat, eggs, nuts, seeds, low-fat milk and yogurt.

Aim to eat a meal or snack within 2 hours of finishing your training session, and drink plenty of fluid – water is good or try diluted fruit juice or an isotonic sports drink. Always plan ahead and carry suitable snacks (see box) in your car's glove compartment, sports bag or briefcase.

Making small changes for big rewards

Improving your diet involves making changes and old habits are always hard to break. Rather than trying to change your diet overnight why not think about one or two changes you can make, see how you get on and then make a couple more when you're ready? For example, at breakfast top your cereal and milk with fresh fruit, opt for wholemeal rather than white bread and try grilled rather than fried bacon, mushrooms and tomatoes. For lunch, add a salad to your meal or choose lean fillings in your sandwiches. At dinner time, opt for fish more often than you used to and add plenty of vegetables. When you want a snack, consider fresh or dried fruit, a handful of peanuts and raisins or a small pot of low-fat yogurt, rice pudding or custard.

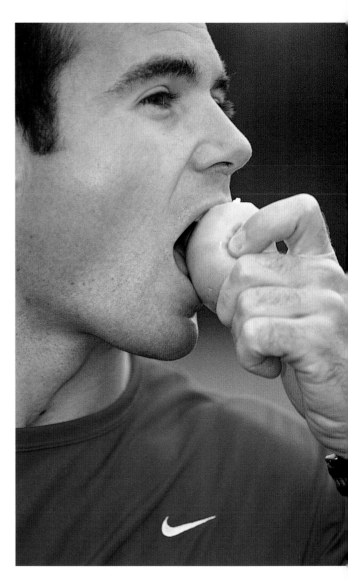

There are no good foods or bad foods, just good and bad diets.

FAQs

Q Do I need to eat more protein when I exercise?

A Yes, but not in the amounts commonly suggested. Your need for protein does rise as a result of exercise but if you eat sufficient amounts of carbohydrate and other foods then you can usually get all the protein you need from your daily diet. There is some evidence to suggest that the timing of protein intake may be important but more research is needed to establish clear guidelines.

Q Is alcohol good for my heart?

A There is evidence to suggest that moderate amounts of alcohol, between one and two units a day (one unit is equivalent to a glass of wine, a measure of spirits or a half pint of beer) can protect against coronary heart disease, but this protection is thought to be significant only for men over the age of 40.

Q Should I take vitamin and mineral supplements?

A Nutritional deficiency in people who have a balanced diet is pretty rare these days and many people who take vitamin and mineral supplements probably do not need to. However, some scientists suggest that men over the age of 65 should take a multi-vitamin and mineral supplement as the body may have a reduced ability to absorb nutrients. If you exclude many foods from your diet, either deliberately or because you eat haphazardly, then you, too, should consider taking a daily multi-vitamin and mineral supplement. However, you should really focus on making a healthy balanced diet your first strategy since supplementation does not make a bad diet better. One exception may be folic acid, which is a B vitamin found in avocado, green leafy vegetables, wholegrains, lentils and orange juice. Folic acid lowers the body's level of an amino acid called homocysteine. High levels of homocysteine have been linked to an increased risk of heart disease.

portable snacks and drinks

A long day at work can wreak havoc on your diet if you don't plan ahead. You can spend the day living on junk food, but if you want to maintain a healthy diet while you are busy, the smart choice is to plan ahead and prepare your food the night before. All it takes is getting into the routine and there will be less chance to make those poor choices.

- Fresh or dried fruit
- Low-fat cereal bar
- Bagel or soft pretzel
- Boxes of raisins
- Nuts and seed mix
- Plain biscuits or crackers
- Bottle of water or isotonic sports drink

a holistic approach

Busy lifestyles mean we often neglect to take care of ourselves and the ensuing stress can manifest itself in many different ways – not just in an inability to sleep but also sports injuries, back pain, poor posture and problems with indigestion.

Taking a holistic approach may be the answer for people who suffer from persistent ailments or injuries, or who would just like to feel better generally. The term 'complementary', or 'alternative', medicine refers to a group of therapeutic and diagnostic disciplines that focus on preventing, alleviating or treating illness and promoting health and wellbeing. The disciplines encompass a variety of health systems and practices with accompanying theories and beliefs, and exist largely outside the confines of conventional healthcare.

If you decide to consult a complementary therapist I strongly recommend that you see one who belongs to a national governing body and who can produce credentials on demand.

complementary therapies

therapy	problems
Acupuncture	Back and neck pain, headaches, skin complaints, sports injuries and insomnia
Ayurveda	Allergies, arthritis and migraines
Homeopathy	Menstrual disorders, allergies, asthma, migraine and eczema
Massage	Poor circulation, stress, fatigue, postural distortions and rheumatism
Naturopathy/ nutrition therapy	Skin disorders, asthma, allergies, arthritis and digestive problems
Reflexology	Migraine, stress, muscular pain, tension and anxiety

Detox

Our bodies are designed to expel toxins naturally, but our modern-day lifestyles and environment tend to overload our bodies with toxins from, for example, pollution, chemical products, a poor diet, stress, drugs, cigarettes and alcohol. Our body systems then struggle to keep up the pace. Detox (short for detoxification) is a systematic approach to assisting the body to remove the toxins from its tissues. There are a great many steps you can take to help your body's natural detox process, for example you could follow a specific detox diet programme set out by a natural therapist. In addition, you can help limit extra stress on your overworked body by making informed decisions that limit your toxic exposure, for example drinking only purified water and eating fresh organic food.

Acupuncture

Acupuncturists believe that if someone's vitality or energy levels are recognizably diminished it is an indication that their organs or tissues are functioning poorly and their flow of *qi*, or *chi*, (energy) is disrupted and inadequate. Acupuncture involves stimulating areas along the 'meridians', the pathways via which *chi* flows through the body, in order to promote healing and good health. An acupuncturist will assess and adjust the flow and distribution by inserting needles into the sufferer's skin at certain specific points along the meridians and leaving them in place for 15–45 minutes, depending on the treatment.

Ayurveda

An ancient healthcare system originating from India, Ayurveda (meaning 'science of life') is based on the principle that disease is the natural end result of living out of harmony with our environment. Ayurveda offers a

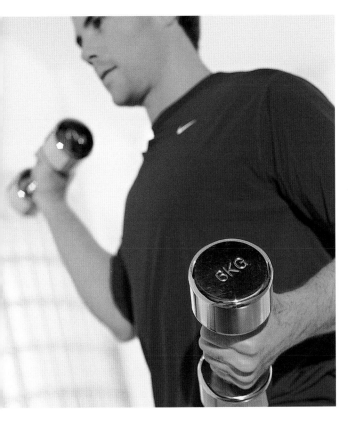

are seen by homeopaths as signs that the vital force is fighting back. Rather than suppress the symptoms, homeopaths prescribe remedies to stimulate this self-healing process.

Massage

Massage is one of the most ancient forms of therapy. It increases circulation throughout the body, helping people to relax and stimulating the workings of various bodily systems. Massage can be used to help the body's muscles regain their correct posture and counteract the effects of stress on everyday life.

Naturopathy/nutrition therapy

Naturopathy is a distinct and total philosophy of life and health that addresses the sick individual as a whole rather than just his or her symptoms. The practitioner emphasizes that the body has the power to heal itself and that illness is a reaction to disharmony and imbalance. The cause could be physical or psychological, but health is regained if nothing interferes with the natural process of healing and recovery. Naturopaths may incorporate other holistic therapies such as osteopathy, homeopathy and herbal therapy.

Reflexology

According to reflexologists, there are pressure, or reflex, points on the feet and hands that correspond directly to a particular function or part of the body. Applying pressure to a specific point on the foot or hand energizes the corresponding zone or function of the body, thereby eliminating toxins and stimulating the body's own healing and balancing processes.

detailed science of diet and herbal therapy, aromatherapy and colour, sound and touch therapy to help clients create an optimal environment for health. Much emphasis is placed on prevention as well as treatment of a huge variety of illnesses, conditions and diseases. Ayurveda incorporates various forms of treatment, including medicines derived from plants and minerals, yoga, meditation, massage, hydrotherapy and diet.

Homeopathy

Homeopathy uses various plants and minerals in very small doses to stimulate a sick person's natural defences. According to homeopathy, if the vital force, the energy, running through the body is below par then illness can occur. Symptoms that appear when we are ill

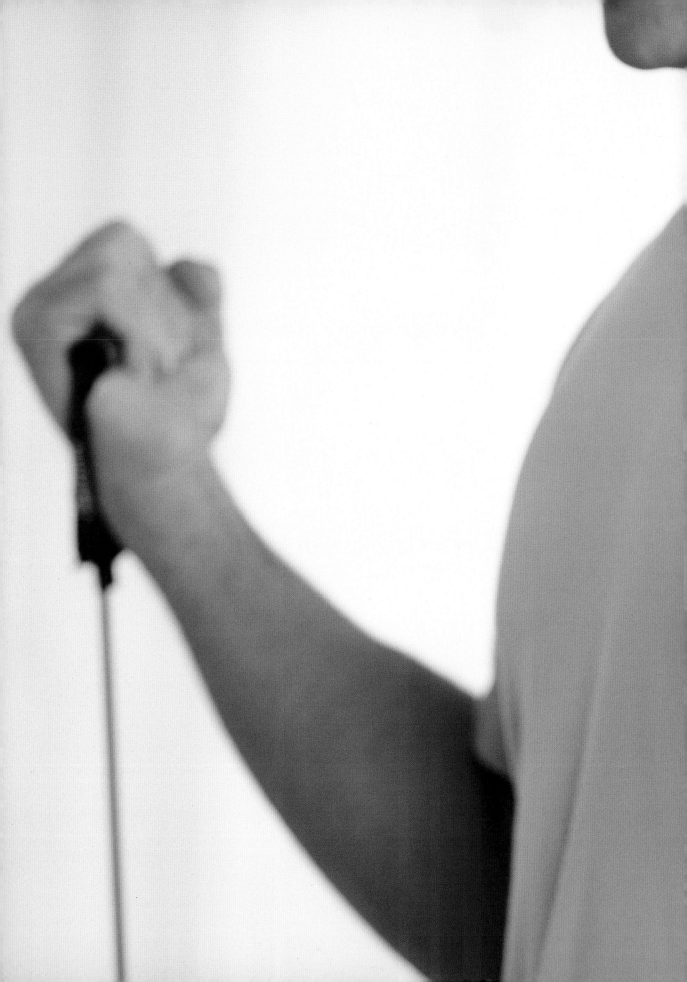

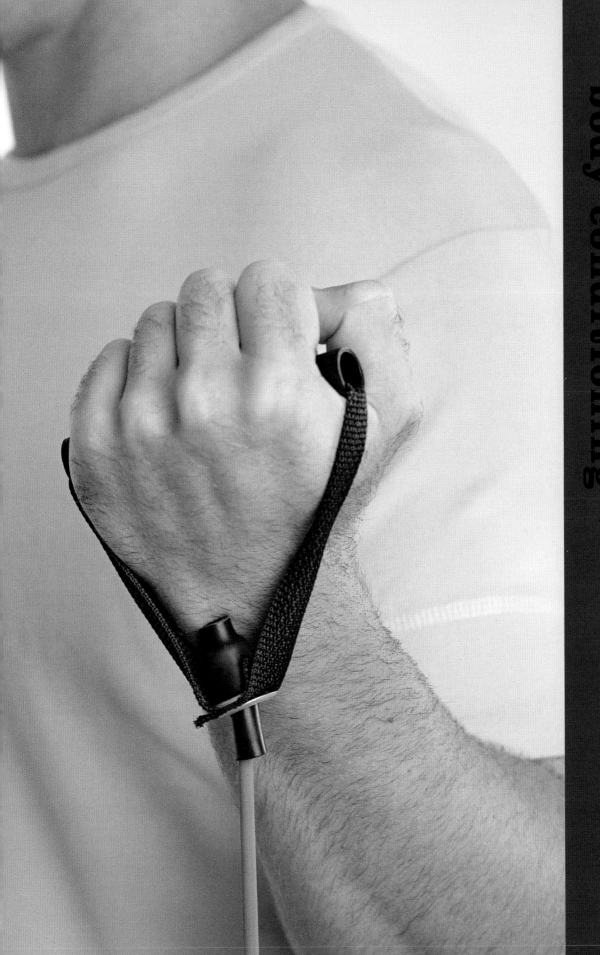

how the programme works

The body conditioning programme relies on the pyramid system, a training method that makes you work progressively harder over the 12 weeks and builds on your achievements at each level to create a strong physical base – like a pyramid. Weeks 1–4 of the programme work on improving your stability, weeks 5–8 concentrate on endurance as well as continuing to work on stability and weeks 9–12 focus on strength in addition to stability and endurance.

The programme is based on functional training and, since the main goal of the programme is for the user to function better physically in general, the skills and strength gained during the programme will transfer well to everyday life. The training programme also follows a progressive exercise philosophy, using various multi-directional and multi-joint movements.

In addition to the pyramid system body conditioning exercises (see pages 32–35), the programme includes exercises to improve your posture and flexibility (see pages 26–31), as well as cardiovascular training (see pages 36–39).

Building a strong base

The body conditioning exercises emphasize the body's stabilizing muscles, including the hip and spine (the core), shoulder and ankle stabilizers. They also work on improving your balance and coordination for the purpose of rehabilitating, stabilizing, protecting and strengthening any weak joints in your body. They utilize full body movements, using the whole body as one system so as to use more muscles at the same time.

The programme tackles the most general of muscular imbalances, commonly caused by past injuries, poor posture or a faulty movement pattern caused by some repeated activity. Muscular imbalances create stress in joints, eventually resulting in compensation by other

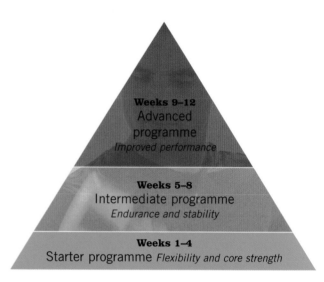

Weeks 9–12
Advanced programme
Improved performance

Weeks 5–8
Intermediate programme
Endurance and stability

Weeks 1–4
Starter programme *Flexibility and core strength*

As you progress through the programme you will be able to build on the initial training and advance to a greater level of intensity, with your body functioning optimally and ultimately performing better.

why do body conditioning?

- Reduce your body fat
- Increase your lean muscle
- Gain strength
- Reduce the risk of injury
- Increase your endurance
- Optimize your flexibility
- Improve performance in your chosen activity

joints and the deterioration of the original joint until there is discomfort and ultimately chronic pain, such as back pain (lower and upper), knee pain, neck pain and headaches.

The programme addresses these issues, incorporating a corrective aspect for posture in its initial stages with a counteractive stretching programme of SMR foam rolling and static stretching so that you can overcome any poor postural habits.

Throughout the body conditioning programme we will concentrate on increasing your strength, while also maintaining stability, removing stress from your joints and getting your muscle system to work the way it is supposed to. The key is to progress within your ability. You are only as strong as you are stable. Building a strong base and correcting muscular imbalances will ensure that your body is prepared for the adaptation to an increase in intensity of exercise and is able to cope without experiencing injury.

The importance of progression

Progressive training is a concept that sometimes gets lost in the exercise arena. Performing new exercises is like taking on any new skill and needs to be mastered at a basic level or a suitable level specifically for you, before moving on to the next degree of intensity. Here are some simple concepts and rules to help you judge your own progression pathway as you work through the body conditioning programme:

Easy to hard The exercise should always start off at an easy level, for example lifting a light weight or performing a simple movement.

Simple to complex Begin with an exercise that is basic and then progress to one of increased complexity.

Known to unknown If possible, use a movement that is more familiar to you that will aid in your ability to execute good form and technique.

Stable to unstable The big push towards what is called functional training in recent years has seen an increase in exercise aids like instability equipment, for example the Swiss ball. You will know if you are working within your limits as you will still be able to control the exercise and have the full range of motion on each movement. Make sure that you are able to complete an exercise on two legs first, before performing the same exercise using just one leg, followed by both legs on an unstable base.

Body weight to loaded Use your body weight only, or a percentage of your weight, as the first stage then increase the intensity of the exercise by adding some other form of resistance like an additional weight.

Slow to fast, or static to dynamic Complete the exercise in a slow fashion before attempting a faster tempo or a dynamic type of movement.

Correct execution to increased intensity Make sure you follow the rule of perfect execution. There is no substitute for consistently good form and technique.

Taking only one step at a time and progressing at a healthy pace will ensure that you are able to move forwards in the programme safely and effectively, ensuring that you don't lose interest in an exercise regime that is too difficult for you to accomplish. Each of the exercises on pages 80–131 has additional information describing how you can make the exercise more difficult and progress to the next level of intensity.

warm-up and cool-down

Warm-up activities are a crucial part of any exercise regime and their importance when it comes to preventing injury and preparing for a good workout should not be underestimated. Similarly, once you have finished any form of physical activity, you should cool down properly, allowing your heart and respiratory rates to gradually drop to a comfortable level, at which you can talk with ease.

Warming up

Warming up prior to any workout does a number of beneficial things, but its main purpose is to prepare the body and mind for more strenuous activity. One of the ways this is achieved is by helping to increase the body's core temperature, while also increasing muscle temperature. This helps to make the muscles loose, supple and pliable.

An effective warm-up also has the effect of increasing both your heart rate and your respiratory rate. This increases blood flow, which in turn increases the speed of delivery of oxygen and nutrients to the working muscles. All this helps to prepare the muscles and tendons for more strenuous activity.

The body conditioning warm-up starts with SMR foam rolling exercises (see pages 44–53). These are followed by static stretching exercises (see pages 56–65) to reset commonly overtight muscles to their normal length, put the body in a better alignment and create the range of motions that you will then need to strengthen and learn to control, Finally there is moderate cardiovascular (CV) exercise – working at about 30–50 per cent of your maximum heart rate (see page 36) – for 5 minutes.

The full warm-up should take 15 minutes in total and should be undertaken before all exercise, even on CV-only training days.

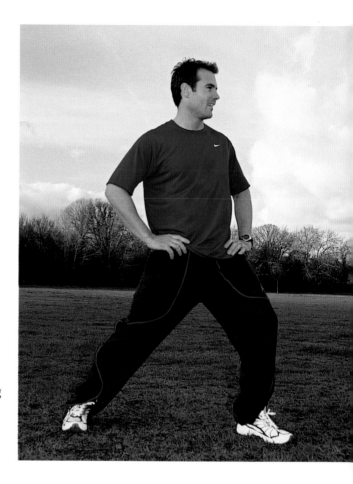

Cooling down

The cool-down helps to reset your muscles after movement. At the end of your workout continue to exercise at about 30–50 per cent of your maximum heart rate for 5 minutes – light aerobic exercises such as walking or easy indoor cycling are good activities for cooling down and aiding your recovery. Follow this with SMR foam rolling and static stretching exercises as for your warm-up. The full cool-down should take 15 minutes in total and, again, you should complete it after all exercise, even on CV-only training days.

15-minute warm-up

SMR foam rolling (see pages 44–53)

Calf

Hamstring

IT band

Quadriceps

Inner thigh

Buttock

Back (lats)

Middle back (rhomboids)

Chest

Static stretching (see pages 56–65)

Calf stretch

Hip and thigh stretch

Inner thigh and lat stretch

Chest stretch

Lat stretch

Front neck stretch

Levator scapulae stretch

Upper trapezius stretch

Back extension with a Swiss ball

Moderate CV exercise (e.g. 5 minutes walking, light jogging, trampolining or indoor cycling)

15-minute cool-down

Moderate CV exercise (e.g. 5 minutes walking, light jogging, trampolining or indoor cycling)

SMR foam rolling (see pages 44–53)

Calf

Hamstring

IT band

Quadriceps

Inner thigh

Buttock

Back (lats)

Middle back (rhomboids)

Chest

Static stretching (see pages 56–65)

Calf stretch

Hip and thigh stretch

Inner thigh and lat stretch

Chest stretch

Lat stretch

Front neck stretch

Levator scapulae stretch

Upper trapezius stretch

Back extension with a Swiss ball

posture

The massive increase in technology in modern society has changed the way we live and work. A high percentage of the workforce now sits at a computer and/or are on the telephone for most of the day. At home, inventions like remote controls, vacuum cleaners and washing machines have reduced the opportunities for physical activity. Our increasingly sedentary lifestyles are resulting both in a decrease in the performance of body systems that were regularly challenged in the past and in poor posture. Our work desks, computers, phones, TVs and cars are shaping our bodies, and shoulders, necks, hips, knees and ankles that are meant to work together are rounded, forwards, elevated, rotated and everted. It is no surprise then that we are seeing rising incidences of, for example, low back pain and joint pain (most of which can be related to poor posture and muscular imbalance), obesity and anterior cruciate ligament injuries among the population.

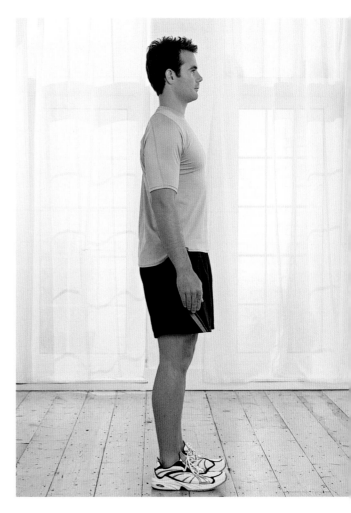

Optimum posture

Posture can be defined as body alignment – it is an indication of your muscle balance, your mechanical efficiency, your body's sense of where it is in space and its ability to coordinate movement. Optimum posture is the balance between the muscles and joints that protect the support systems of the body against injury and progressive deformity, both during movement and at rest.

Good postural habits begin with self-awareness. Notice how you stand, walk, sit, work at your desk and talk on the telephone. If you are tired, stiff or stressed at the end of the day, you need to adopt the following good habits to ensure good posture:

- Lift objects by bending at your knees instead of your back, using your leg and stomach muscles to do the lifting.

common causes of poor posture

- Poor postural habits at rest (sitting or standing) and in motion (running, walking, lifting, etc.)
- Psychological (self-esteem or stress)
- Normal developmental and degenerative processes
- Pain leading to muscle guarding and avoidance postures
- Muscle imbalance or spasm
- Respiratory conditions
- General weakness and deconditioning, i.e. the core
- Obesity

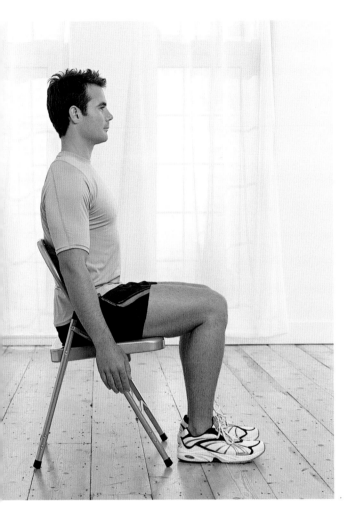

• Vary your workout routines.

• Try having a sports massage to help break down knots that can affect flexibility and posture.

• Get plenty of sleep.

• Maintain your ideal body weight.

• Get a postural assessment from a qualified movement screening specialist so that a corrective postural-specific programme can be created for you.

Assessing and correcting your posture

Over time postural and structural changes can occur, for example certain muscles may become weaker and longer. These changes can alter a muscle's mechanical line and/or lines of pull and may cause other muscles and muscle groups to compensate, thereby directly altering the mechanics of your joints. This alteration or compensation leads to a decrease in performance and a risk of injury, and may result in inflammatory responses to overstressed joints, lower back pain, nerve impingements, ligament laxity or muscle spasms.

I have included within my body conditioning programme corrective exercises – SMR foam rolling (see pages 29 and 44–53) and static stretching (see pages 56–65) – to cater for the most common postural problems. By performing these you can improve your posture, flexibility, muscle function and performance, reduce injuries and shorten your recovery time after exercising. However, you may find it necessary to consult a professional for assistance in creating a personal programme tailored to your own needs. An assessment of your posture by a qualified movement screening professional or exercise specialist will evaluate your body's mechanical connections and allow the results to be incorporated into your exercise programme, thereby making it even more specific and ensuring an injury-free response to your training.

• Carry objects close to your body, switching arms often. Try to use a backpack rather than a shoulder bag.

• To counter the effects of constant sitting, frequently vary from sitting to standing, or stand and stretch periodically throughout the day.

• During resistance exercise, alternate pressing and pulling movements evenly to avoid the risk of muscular imbalance.

• Hold the telephone to your ear with your hand not your shoulder or use a hands-free set.

• Adjust the seat in your car so that you do not have to reach for the steering wheel.

precaution

Consult a healthcare provider before taking up foam rolling, particularly if you suffer from any deficiency/condition in the body, which causes bruising from any kind of pressure. Be cautious when rolling near areas like the ribs as direct body weight pressure may cause injury. Using the foam roll for other than its recommended use may cause injury.

SMR and stretches for postural distortion

Pelvis and hips (lower crossed syndrome)	Ankles (pronation distortion syndrome)	Neck and shoulders (upper crossed syndrome)
Calf (see pages 44–45)	Calf (see pages 44–45)	Back (see pages 50–51)
Hamstring (see pages 46–47)	Hamstring (see pages 46–47)	Middle back (see page 52–53)
IT band (see page 47)	Buttocks (see page 50)	Lat stretch (see page 60)
Quadriceps (see page 48)	Calf stretch (see pages 56–57)	Chest (see page 53)
Inner thigh (see page 49)		Levator scapulae stretch (see page 62)
Buttocks (see page 50)		Front neck stretch (see pages 62–63)
Calf stretch (see pages 56–57)		Upper trapezius stretch (see page 65)
Inner thigh and lat stretch (see pages 58–59)		Back extension with Swiss ball (see page 64–65)
Hip and thigh stretch (see page 59)		

Postural distortion patterns

A postural distortion pattern is when the body adopts a pattern of movement that does not use the muscle in an optimum fashion, thereby causing altered muscle function and possible injury. There are three main areas in the body where postural distortion patterns commonly occur – the ankles (pronation distortion syndrome), the pelvis and hips (lower crossed syndrome) and the neck and shoulders (upper crossed syndrome). If you experience one of these distortion patterns, the problem can be addressed with SMR foam rolling and some key stretches (see left) in order for you to follow the body conditioning programme successfully.

SMR foam rolling

SMR foam rolling is a form of stretching that is a precursor to a true stretch. It involves you using your own body weight to roll on a foam roll to massage away knots and help return muscles to their normal length-tension relationship (see the exercises, pages 44–53).

To truly understand the 'magic' of SMR (self-myofascial release) foam rolling you need a basic understanding of the muscular system, also known as the kinetic chain. The kinetic chain is made up of the soft tissue system (muscles, tendons, ligaments and fascia), the central nervous system (nerves) and the articular system (joints). These systems work together as a unit – if one system is not functioning efficiently, then the others must compensate. This can lead to tissue overload, fatigue, faulty movement patterns, poor posture and recurring injury. For example a tight muscle will restrict how much a joint can move; over time you become accustomed to moving in that way and adopt a poor movement or posture, resulting in an injury.

When the body is injured it is prone to lay down tissue to strengthen the area. The tissue is laid in criss-cross patterns much like the plys of a tyre, forming 'knots', or adhesions. The best way to get rid of these adhesions is through SMR massage with the foam roll.

How does it work?

The SMR foam roll will allow you to identify muscle tension in the area where it is being used, often appearing as a 'sore' or 'tight' spot. SMR foam rolling will enhance the release of the tension, allowing the muscle to return to its correct length. You may find the foam rolling uncomfortable, not unlike a strong sports massage. Foam rolling is most effective when followed by the correct flexibility procedure for that muscle group, for example a quadriceps foam roll (see page 48) followed by a hip and thigh stretch (see page 59).

The more times you use the foam roll, the fewer tight spots you will experience and the lower the intensity of discomfort. Note that it is important to breathe correctly and concentrate on relaxing when using the foam roll in order to benefit fully from the process. Adhere to the following guidelines:

- Perform the SMR foam roll programme once or twice daily, or before and after a workout. Also do it to break up long periods of sitting, for example at work or before and after aeroplane flights.
- If you find a knot, stop rolling and rest on the tender area for 20–30 seconds.
- Maintain a proper drawn-in position (draw your navel towards your spine for a good postural alignment) so as to stabilize your core when rolling (see 'SMR foam rolling exercises', pages 44–53).

flexibility

Flexibility training is one of the main components of health and fitness. It is as important as cardiovascular training and strength training, although it is often neglected. Without flexibility our bodies can become stiff, our posture less than ideal, our muscles imbalanced and our joints prone to pain and injury.

Some people are naturally more flexible. Flexibility is primarily influenced by one's genetics, gender, age and level of physical activity. As we grow older, we tend to lose flexibility – usually as a result of inactivity rather than the ageing process itself. The less active we are, the less flexible we are likely to be. Like cardiovascular endurance and muscle strength, flexibility will improve with regular training.

With flexibility training, as with any form of exercise, you need to pay equal attention to form, alignment and technique. It is possible to cheat a stretch and create relative flexibility where the body compensates to create movement. Stretching can also progress in the same way that other exercises can. Static, active and dynamic stretching are three of the most common stretching techniques used in a modern progressive flexibility programme. This programme uses both static and active stretching techniques to help correct any potential muscle imbalances right from the start.

Static stretching

Static, or passive, stretching is the process of passively taking a muscle to the point of tension and holding the stretch for 20–30 seconds to allow the soft tissue to be elongated. This style of stretching combines low force movements with long duration. It is the form of stretching most often seen in fitness venues. It should be used to release a tight muscle before activity and to 'reset' your muscles into balance following activity. Make sure you adhere to the following guidelines:

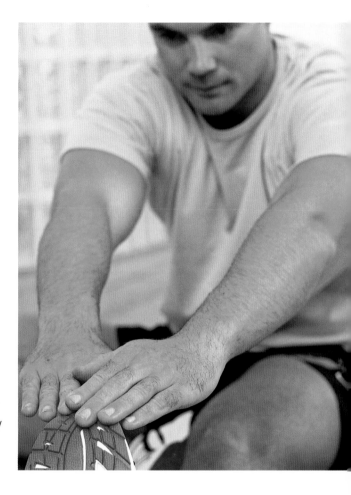

Warm-up Use SMR foam rolling, flexibility training and light to moderate CV exercise to get the best results (see page 24).

Duration and frequency Make stretching a big part of your weekly exercise programme. Try to incorporate flexibility training for the major muscle groups two or three times a week. As far as duration is concerned, the more attention you give to flexibility training the more you will achieve. Spending 15–20 minutes on a quality flexibility programme will give you good results.

Variety There are many tools you can use to enhance your routine, including foam rollers and Swiss balls.

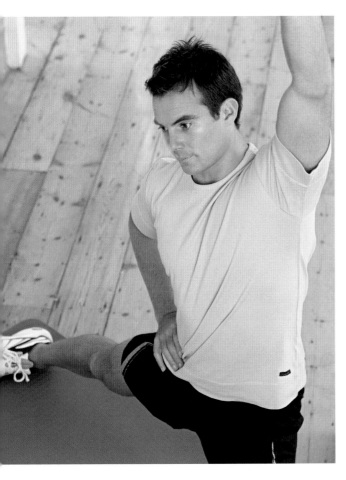

Join a class Yoga and Pilates are two forms of exercise that utilize different stretching techniques to increase flexibility. Joining a class means that you will have an instructor to watch you and teach you the proper technique so that you do not injure yourself.

Pay attention to your posture Not only can you overstretch a muscle, but you can stretch the wrong muscle through common postural distortion patterns (see pages 28–29) and muscular imbalances. Follow the stretching exercises on pages 56–75 properly and you will generally avoid stretching the most common chronically lengthened muscles, and so reduce the chances of injury and pain to that muscle.

Don't overdo it Listen to your body. Stretch slowly and only to first resistance (the point at which the stretch takes hold). Stretching should help reduce the chance of injury, not cause injury.

Active stretching

Once your body has started to adapt and improve its flexibility, you can progress to active stretching. Active stretching uses movement to reteach the body to make use of its flexibility. The basic principles of listening to your body and not overpushing yourself still apply.

The less active we are, the less flexible we are likely to be. Like cardiovascular endurance and muscle strength, however, flexibility will improve with regular training.

benefits of stretching

- Allows greater freedom of movement and improved posture
- Increases physical and mental relaxation
- Releases muscle tension and soreness
- Reduces risk of injury

the exercises

The body conditioning programme is designed to stimulate many of the body's different capabilities. The exercises therefore focus on core stability, balance, reaction time and strength. These four elements together comprise a truly functional and complete approach to body conditioning.

Core training

The hottest fitness trend to hit the gyms of late, core training includes any exercise that works the pelvic girdle, the deep abdominal muscles often ignored by other exercise programmes. These muscles in particular have a starring role in maintaining your posture and are crucial in the stabilization of the lower spine, because they surround it like a snug muscular corset. Recommended by sport scientists, physiotherapists and osteopaths, core stability is the new fitness buzzword that is a part of the latest fitness advances.

Core stabilization is the foundation upon which all other aspects of training are based. Your core is made up of the muscles of the torso that are engaged in supporting the trunk and spine. Core training involves performing an exercise or using equipment like the Swiss ball to put the body in a controlled unstable position, thereby requiring it to activate its stabilizing system to maintain balance. In other words you are working your core!

The purposes of core training are to strengthen the muscle groups that stabilize your skeletal structure and to maintain the balance throughout the body's muscular chain. The state of your core determines your posture in everyday life and during activity and, in effect, links your upper and lower body. The muscle groups that you strengthen with core training form the 'platform' from which your arms and legs work. In an out-of-condition body it is likely that the core is not functioning optimally. It will be stimulated when you draw your navel towards your spine, which is why this action is the starting point for many of the exercises throughout the book and should be held for the duration of the exercise.

Balance training

Balance training is simply defined as challenging your balance. Whether you are a hitting a golf ball, exercising on a Swiss ball or walking down the street, maintaining your balance is the key to movement. In everyday activities balance does not work just by itself so it should not be regarded as an isolated component of real-life movements. Balance is a component of all movements; regardless of whether you are doing strength, flexibility or endurance training, it dominates the exercise because without it we cannot move.

It therefore makes sense to practise an aspect of balance in an exercise programme so that it can be improved upon and help the performance of other activities, even if this is only to function better in everyday life. Some of the exercises in this book require use of a Swiss ball to practise balance, others simply involve standing on one leg.

Reactive training

Reactive, or power, training is defined as a quick, powerful movement involving an eccentric contraction followed immediately by an explosive concentric contraction, for example the crouched position in preparation for a tuck jump then the actual jump itself. Such an exercise helps the body decelerate and stabilize when you land.

Reactive training is vital if your other training only uses muscle contraction, such as swimming, working on a treadmill or cycling, as you need to train your body's decelerators.

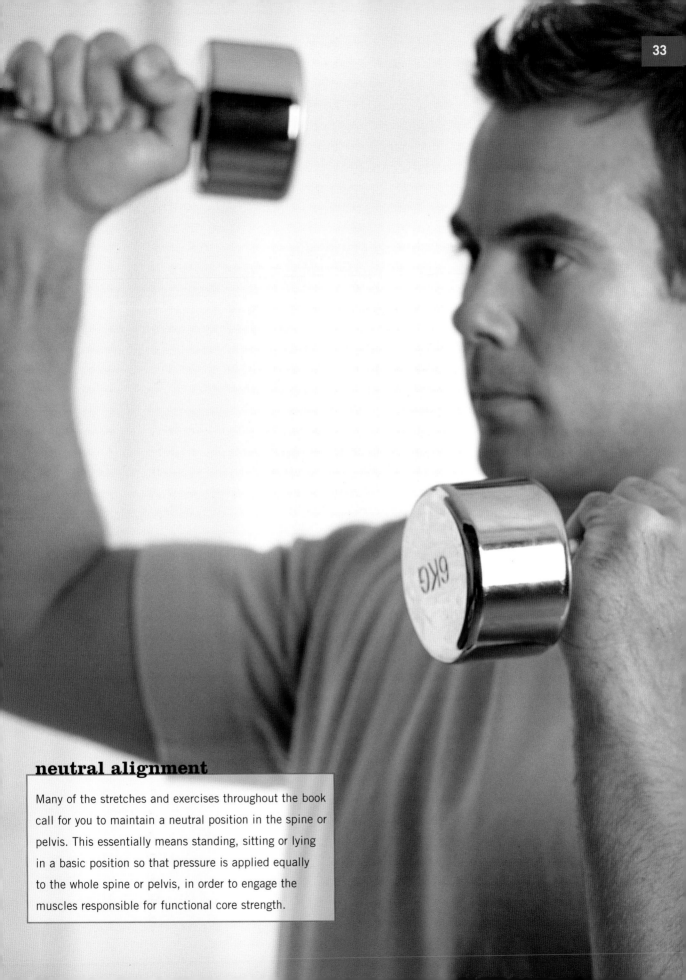

neutral alignment

Many of the stretches and exercises throughout the book
call for you to maintain a neutral position in the spine or
pelvis. This essentially means standing, sitting or lying
in a basic position so that pressure is applied equally
to the whole spine or pelvis, in order to engage the
muscles responsible for functional core strength.

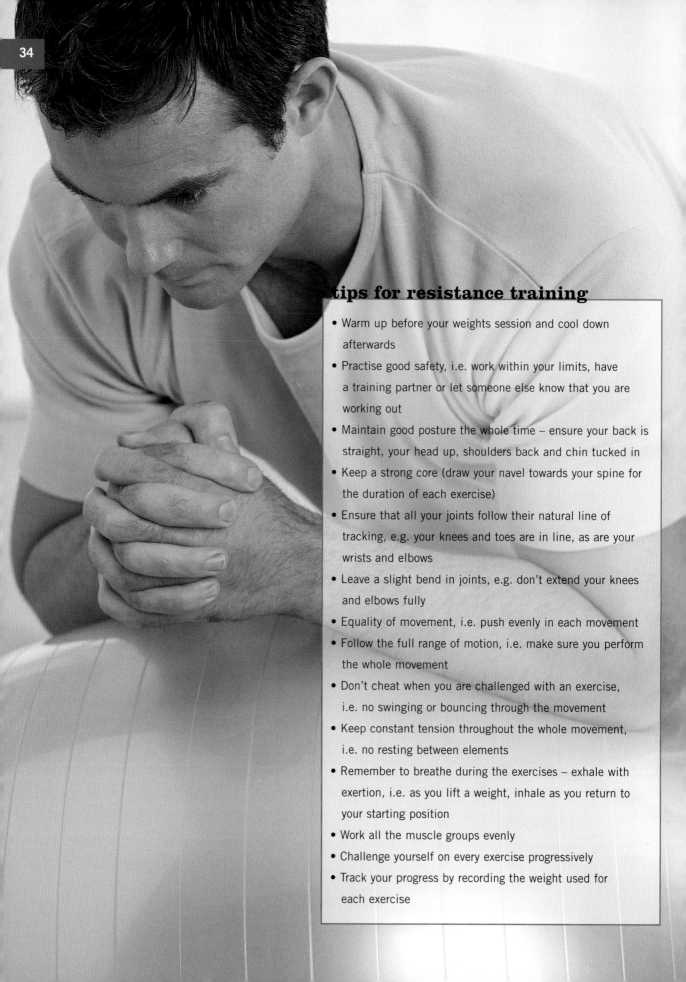

tips for resistance training

- Warm up before your weights session and cool down afterwards
- Practise good safety, i.e. work within your limits, have a training partner or let someone else know that you are working out
- Maintain good posture the whole time – ensure your back is straight, your head up, shoulders back and chin tucked in
- Keep a strong core (draw your navel towards your spine for the duration of each exercise)
- Ensure that all your joints follow their natural line of tracking, e.g. your knees and toes are in line, as are your wrists and elbows
- Leave a slight bend in joints, e.g. don't extend your knees and elbows fully
- Equality of movement, i.e. push evenly in each movement
- Follow the full range of motion, i.e. make sure you perform the whole movement
- Don't cheat when you are challenged with an exercise, i.e. no swinging or bouncing through the movement
- Keep constant tension throughout the whole movement, i.e. no resting between elements
- Remember to breathe during the exercises – exhale with exertion, i.e. as you lift a weight, inhale as you return to your starting position
- Work all the muscle groups evenly
- Challenge yourself on every exercise progressively
- Track your progress by recording the weight used for each exercise

The reactive training exercises form a progression that can be incorporated into a training programme to emulate real-life situations. They enhance the sensitivity and reactivity of the neuromuscular system and help increase the performance of the muscular system. Reactive training is an optional part of this programme, to be used depending on your physical ability.

Resistance training

The terms 'weight training/lifting' and 'strength training' are often used to describe working the muscles by using weights, machines and even your own body weight to work your muscles effectively. Resistance training is the umbrella term used to describe all forms of resistance training, whether working with weights or not. Although strength training accurately describes what resistance training does, many people dislike the term because they think it applies only to those who are trying to become bigger and stronger. In fact, all resistance training when done correctly increases strength, but does not necessarily visibly increase size. Resistance training has received a bad name because of isolated training for mass gain, whereas the goal of the body conditioning programme is to train multi-joints (more than one muscle group) and muscle strength using the new range of motion created in the flexibility training part of the programme. Resistance training can be done by anyone. It is not just for people who are athletes, who want to build or tone muscle or who want to achieve a better looking body.

Resistance training does improve the look and tone of the body but it is now known to be more than just a specialized exercise activity. Medical research has shown that resistance training:
- Strengthens the musculoskeletal system
- Improves bone density and posture
- Increases metabolism and circulation
- Limits atrophy (break-down) of the muscles
- Helps control hypertension, cholesterol and body fat
- Helps prevent heart disease, adult-onset diabetes and certain cancers
- Improves mood, self-esteem and quality of life

These are just a few of the many benefits of resistance training that are well documented by medical professionals. A resistance training programme should be a part of everyone's health and fitness lifestyle, regardless of age, gender or training goals.

Resistance training can be done anywhere and without specialized equipment. You do not have to join a health club or spend a lot of money to do it. You can do resistance training using a home work-out kit.

training terms

Rep A single completed exercise movement

Set A group of reps together (between 12 and 15)

Intensity Measured in one repetition max, this is the greatest amount of weight a person can lift at one time in good form

Tempo The amount of time each repetition takes, for example the time taken to push out a weight, hold it at the top and control the return to the starting position

Rest interval The time taken between each exercise, or set of exercises, usually about 30–90 seconds

Duration The length of the workout, excluding the warm-up, cool-down and CV workout, normally 35–45 minutes in the body conditioning programme

Frequency The number of times the workout is undertaken in a week, ideally three times a week

cardiovascular training

Cardiovascular (CV) training is a vital aspect of any balanced exercise programme. Put simply, it is any training that places a stress on your cardiovascular system (your heart and lungs). Walking, cycling, boxing, rope skipping, trampolining, rowing, running, swimming and using a cross-trainer fitness machine are all examples of CV exercise. You should do any one or more of these activities for 30 minutes as the CV component of the body conditioning programme.

Training heart rate

Your training heart rate zone is an important element of CV exercise as it helps determine the intensity level at which you should work out and whether the exercise is safe and specific to your needs. A heart rate monitor, a transmitter strapped to the chest to record and transmit precise measurements of the heart rate, is one of the many ways in which you can check the intensity level at which you and your heart are working.

To work out your training heart rate zone first calculate your maximum heart rate – in beats per minute (bpm) – by subtracting your age from 220. As a general rule, you should exercise at an intensity level between 50 and 85 per cent of your maximum heart rate. Your individual level of fitness will ultimately determine where you fall within this range:

- **Beginner or low level** 50–60 per cent maximum heart rate
- **Average level** 60–70 per cent maximum heart rate
- **High level** 70–85 per cent maximum heart rate

CV exercise frequency

How often you do CV exercise depends on your goals and time constraints. To improve CV fitness and to keep your body fat at healthy levels, you should aim to do exercise (such as walking, mowing the lawn or even running) five times a week. This can be a cumulative amount of time throughout the day, for example three 10-minute sessions. Three to six times a week may be necessary to lose body fat. Three times a week is appropriate for most beginners following starter programme in weeks 1–4. Excessively overweight beginners who choose weight-bearing exercise such as walking and skipping should rest at least 36–48 hours between sessions to promote adequate bone-stress recovery and prevent overtraining.

The CV aspect of the programme can be tackled immediately after the body conditioning exercises or on a totally separate day, depending on the time you have available. If the CV is done on a different day make sure you still follow the warming up and cooling down programmes (see pages 24–25).

CV exercise intensity

Before beginning the body conditioning programme, you must decide on the intensity level that is most appropriate and effective for you. Exercise intensity is described as the speed and/or workload (calorific cost) of a workout. If you are a beginner and entering the body conditioning programme at the starter level or you currently exercise at a low CV fitness level, low to moderate intensity (50–65 per cent of maximum heart rate) is considered a safe, effective starting point.

benefits of CV training

Decreases Risk of coronary artery disease, cancer, hypertension, osteoporosis and diabetes; and likelihood of obesity, daily fatigue, anxiety and stress

Increases Immune system efficiency, favourable body composition, daily performance – at work and recreation, and sense of wellbeing

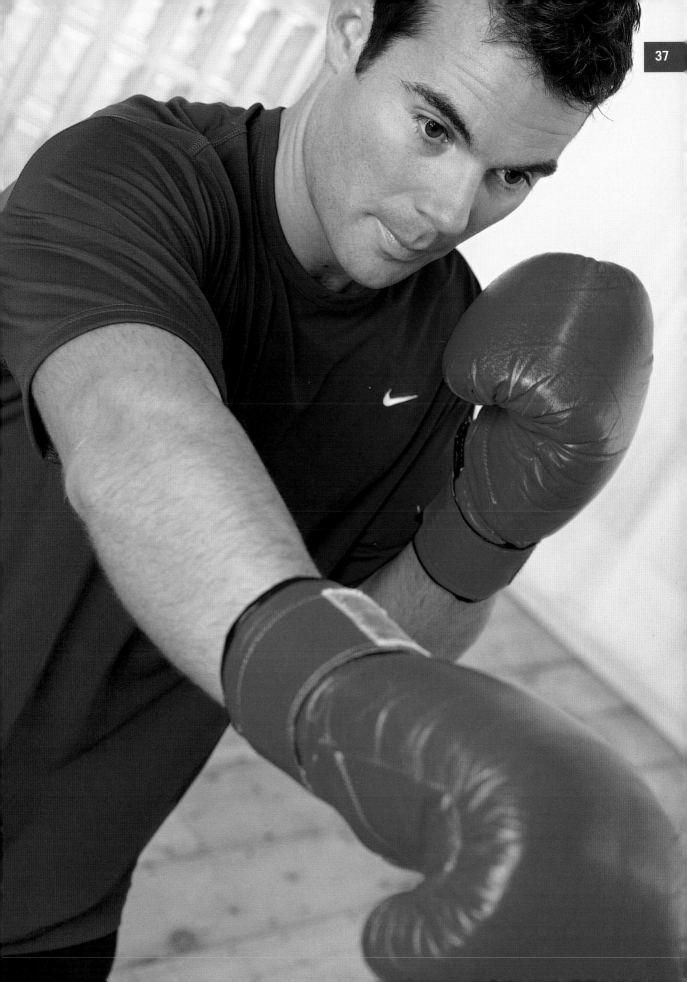

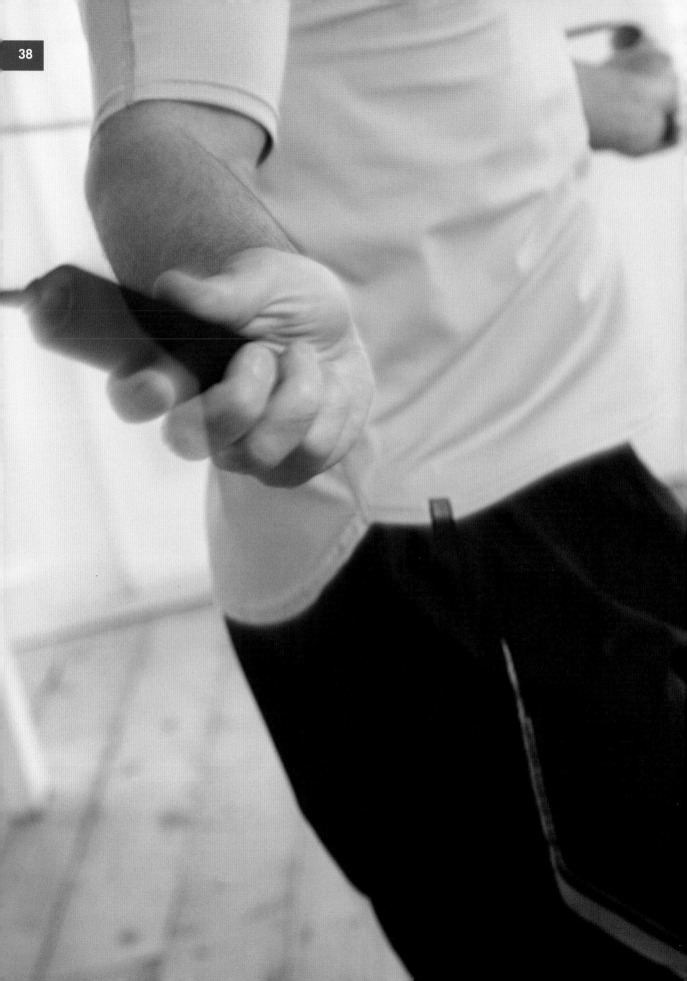

If your goal is to decrease body fat, you should aim to progress to a higher CV intensity level (60–85 per cent of maximum heart rate) in the intensive programme in weeks 9–12.

Interval training

As opposed to normal steady state intensity in a CV exercise programme, interval training allows you to work at a heart rate level much higher than normal but for short interval periods. For example over a 30-minute workout you might work for 1 minute at 60 per cent of your maximum heart rate, then the following minute at 85 per cent. You would continue this for the whole 30 minutes, effectively spending half of the workout at a much higher level of intensity than you would normally be able to sustain for extended periods.

Interval training presents the body with a workload that challenges its current fitness state. This workload will cause temporary fatigue but, the proper recovery, will eventually bring about improvements in both your fitness and your body composition. If the workloads are of the right degree – slightly more than the body is currently used to – then your body will adapt to them. It is important to note that the exercise overload happens during the exercise, and the body recovers and benefits from it during recovery, thus making recovery (see pages 40–41) a vital part of your exercise programme.

Interval training has three important benefits: increased metabolism, increased CV fitness levels and improved motivation:

Increased metabolism An important factor to consider is not only how many calories you burn during your workout, but what your body is doing during the rest of the day. Studies have shown that interval training raises your metabolism after a workout and keeps it up for

longer than any 'steady state' workout (exercise that stays at the same workload for a long period of time, like an aerobics class or normal cycle ride).

Increased cardiovascular system capabilities By overloading the heart and lungs, you increase your endurance and CV fitness level. This is the same principle as weight training where overloading a muscle will result in increasing the strength of the muscle. The heart is a muscle so it, too, must be overloaded to improve its strength. At the same time, the rest of the respiratory system including the lungs and blood circulation improves, resulting in better endurance.

The motivational factor This occurs when you start designing your workouts; the programmes are always changing so you are less likely to experience boredom while performing them.

Summary

All CV exercise is effective for increasing calorific expenditure and helping to lose body fat. It is the intensity of the workout, for example whether you exercise for a longer period of time at a low intensity or for a shorter period at a higher intensity that will affect the speed of your results. High-intensity exercise is an excellent way to break a fat-loss plateau but you must be in good cardiovascular and musculoskeletal (postural) condition before beginning such a workout programme. High-intensity CV activity is not recommended for people who are generally out-of-condition.

The important thing is that you incorporate the 'fun factor' in your workout and choose the CV activity and intensity that suits you. If you don't enjoy your CV workout you are less likely to exercise regularly and stick with the programme.

rest and recovery

Rest and recovery are often the most neglected parts of a training programme. Muscles, joints and connective tissue rebuild and grow stronger on the days that you rest. Rest is therefore very important so that you don't suffer from overtraining. Compare overtraining with a pendulum that swings too far one way – it will inevitably swing back in the opposite direction. In the same way, training too often could cause injury and illness, resulting in downtime from your programme. It puts great stress on your immune system, increasing your chances of becoming sick, and raises your chances of injuring joints such as wrists, elbows and knees.

Overtraining

A little exercise is good for you, so more must be better, right? Well, sometimes, but there comes a point of diminishing returns or, worse, a point where your body says enough!

Everyone reaches this point at different times. Triathletes, for example, are able to withstand the rigours of three-sport training – running, cycling and swimming – at levels unthinkable to most. For others, an extra fitness class or progressing with the weights too fast can put them over the top. In the quest for better health and fitness, it is sometimes difficult to quell one's enthusiasm and take a break from exercise. But if exercise is leaving you more exhausted than energized, you could be suffering from an acute case of overtraining. It's important to be able to recognize the signs of overtraining before they become chronic (see box).

Be aware that not all of the signs of overtraining are physical. Just as regular exercise has a positive effect on mood and stress levels, too much exercise can do the opposite, leaving the exerciser feeling irritable and depressed, particularly as the quality of the workouts declines. Psychological and emotional signs of overtraining include depression, apathy, difficulty concentrating, emotional sensitivity and a reduced sense of self-esteem.

Once you recognize the symptoms of overtraining, it's important to understand and confront the cause honestly. For some people, it occurs as a result of an upcoming competition. Increased training prior to an event is understandable, but if it's interfering with your health and wellbeing, you have to question its worth. The solution to overtraining may be as easy as reducing the rate at which you increase your training intensity. The body needs sufficient time to adjust to your increased demands. Elite triathletes certainly don't start out running 10 miles, cycling 100 miles and swimming 1 kilometre all at once. They gradually increase their training to allow their bodies to adapt.

Addicted to exercise?

The basis for overtraining may have more to do with emotional or psychological reasons than physical ones. Like eating disorders, exercise addiction is now recognized as a legitimate problem. Exercising beyond the point of exhaustion, while injured, or to the exclusion of all other aspects of one's life are some of the signs of exercise addiction. It's a difficult problem

physical signs of overtraining

- Decreased performance
- Loss of coordination
- Prolonged recovery
- Elevated morning heart rate
- Headaches
- Loss of appetite
- Muscle soreness/tenderness
- Decreased ability to ward off infection

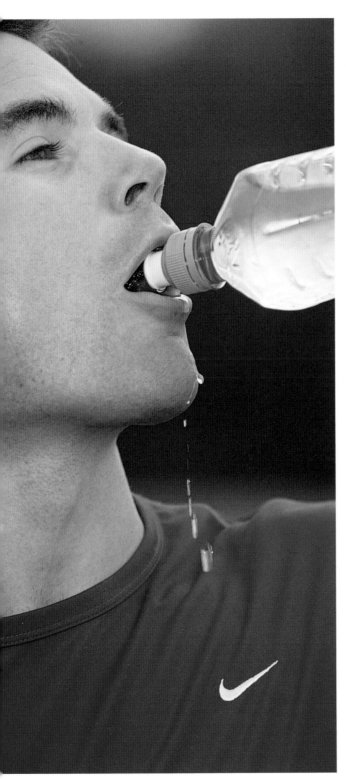

to recognize, particularly in a culture where discipline and control are lauded. Individuals who exercise excessively risk more than poor performance – they risk their health. Overuse syndrome, which may lead to more serious injuries, is common. In addition, the emotional cost of isolating oneself in order to exercise can be devastating. If you recognize these symptoms in yourself or in a friend, it is essential to seek professional help.

Moderation

The key, it seems, to staying healthy is to do everything in moderation, which is best viewed as something relative to one's own fitness level and goals. Don't expect to exercise an hour every day simply because your very fit friend does. The body needs time to adjust, adapt and, yes, even recuperate. Exercising to the point of overtraining is simply taking one step forwards, two steps backwards.

You become fitter when you rest. Your body has a chance to recover and repair and will change and adapt to your specific programme with the result that you achieve your goals.

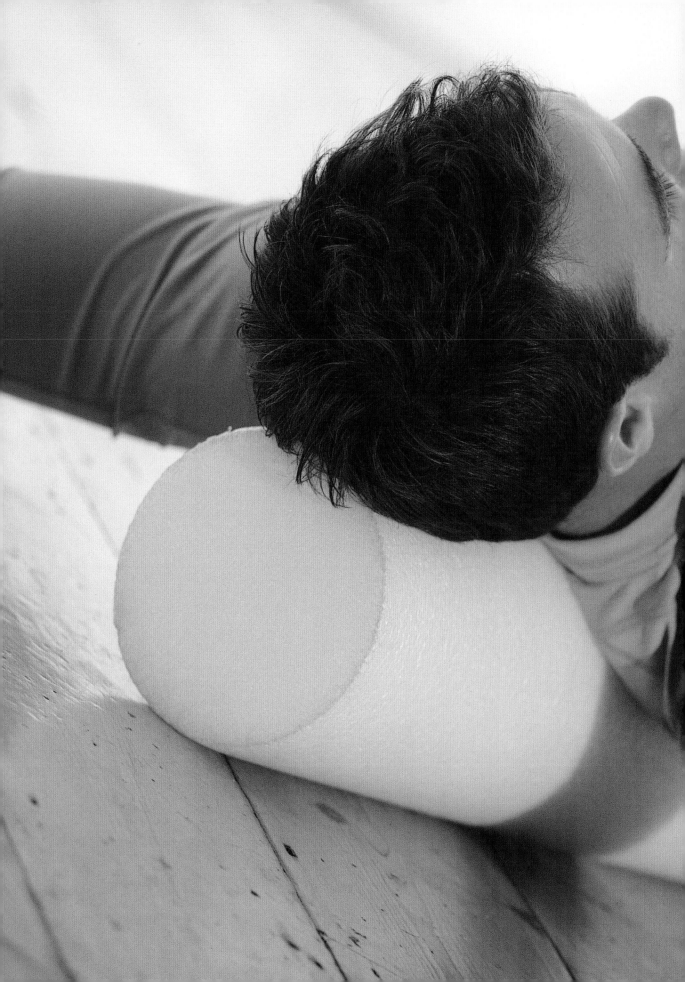

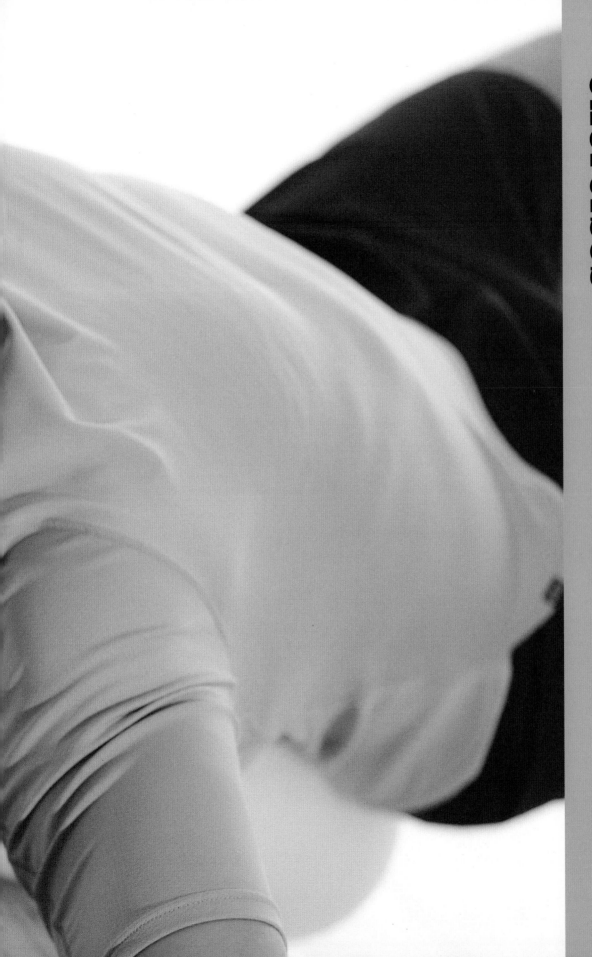

foam rolling
exercises

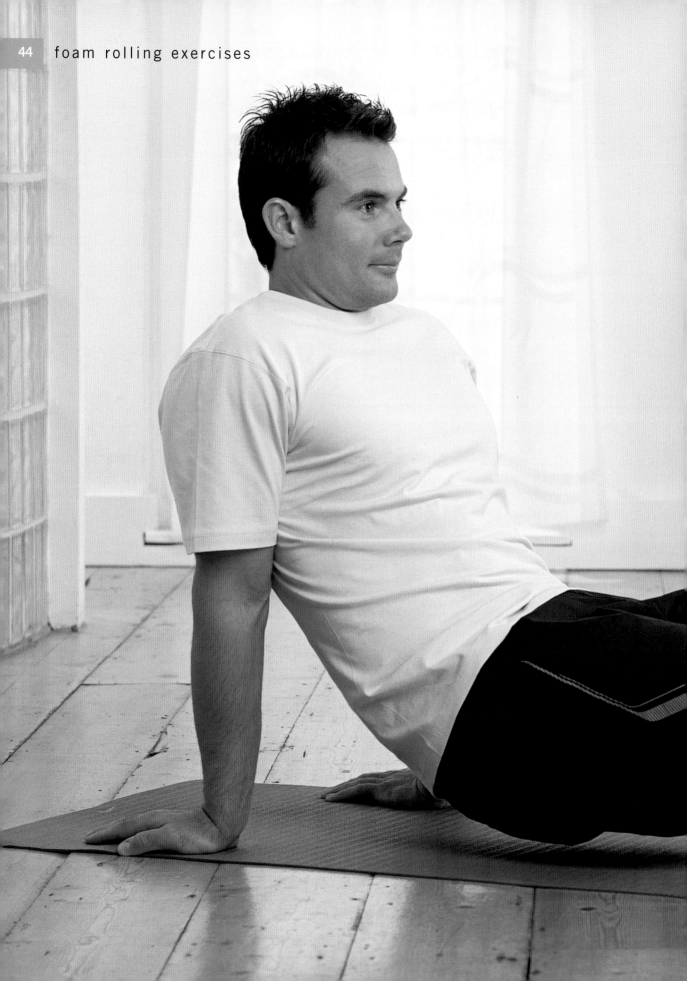

calf

SMR (self-myofascial release) foam rolling is a form of stretching, which in conjunction with static stretching exercises can help improve your posture and flexibility (see page 30). The exercises should also form a part of every warm-up and cool-down session. The simple technique of SMR foam rolling can be performed almost anywhere – at home, at the gym, in your hotel room after a long flight or even in your coffee break at work. Make sure you pay particular attention to your form and technique so that the exercises have the optimum effect on your body.

Sit on the floor, your legs stretched out in front of you and place the foam roll under the back of one knee. (An optional extra for harder rolling is to cross your opposite leg over the top of the leg that is being rolled, resting it on your shin to increase the pressure.) Support your body with your hands placed flat on the floor behind you and raise your buttocks off the mat. Slowly roll down the calf to find the tender area, emphasizing the muscle belly of the lower leg area. To explore the whole calf muscle roll your foot inwards and outwards, hitting both sides of the muscle. If a 'tender point' is located, stop rolling and rest on the tender point for 20–30 seconds. Repeat on the other side.

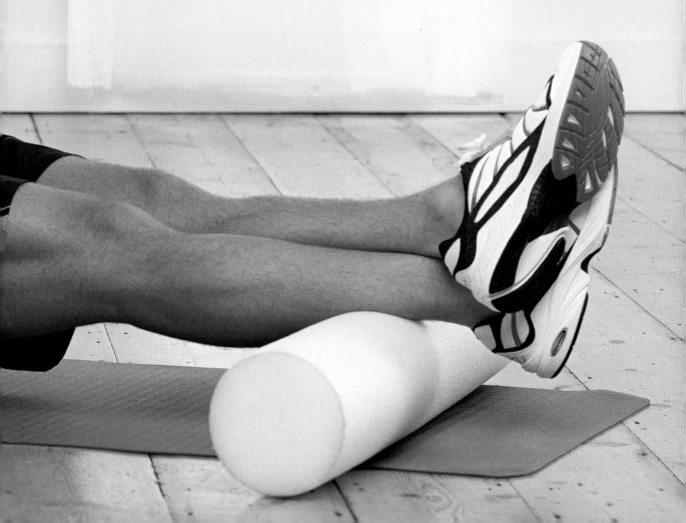

hamstring

1 Sit on the floor, your legs stretched out in front of you and place the foam roll under the back of one thigh (the hamstring) just above the back of the knee. (An optional extra for harder rolling is to cross your opposite leg over the top of the leg that is being rolled, resting it on your shin to increase the pressure.) Support your body with your hands placed flat on the floor behind you and raise your buttocks off the mat.

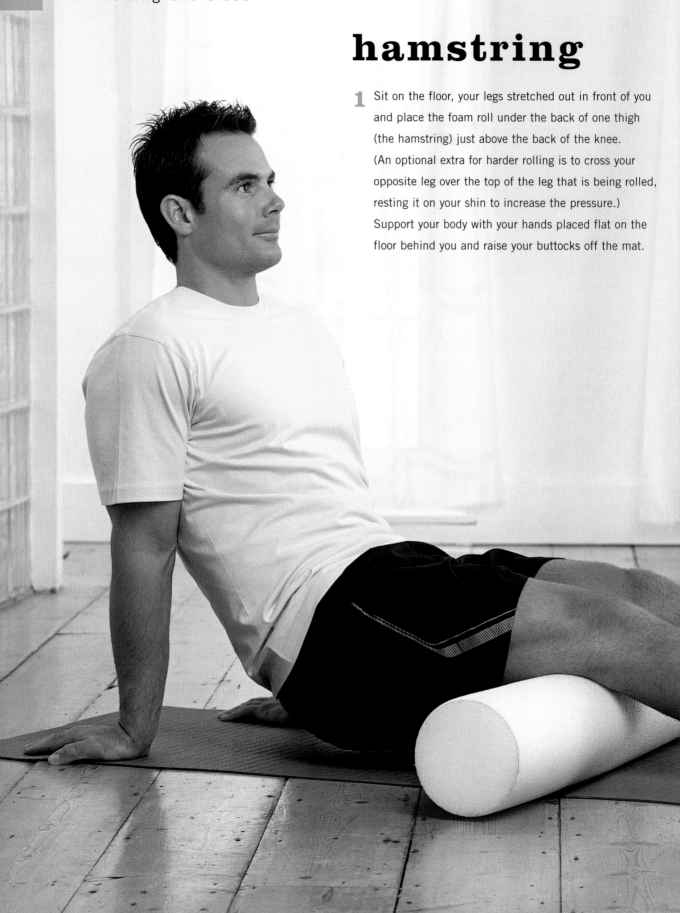

IT band

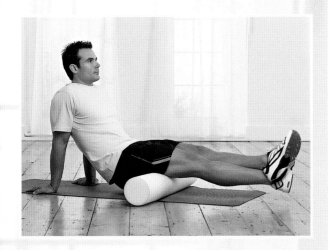

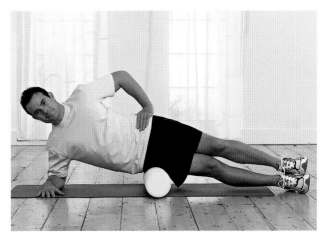

2 Slowly roll the foam up the hamstring, finishing at the crease where the leg meets the buttocks. If a 'tender point' is located, stop rolling and rest on the tender point for 20–30 seconds. Repeat on the other side.

1 The IT (iliotibial tract) band is the side of your upper leg, from the hip to the knee. Lie on your side on the floor with the foam roll beneath your hip. Maintain good body alignment throughout, drawing your navel towards your spine to prevent poor posture.

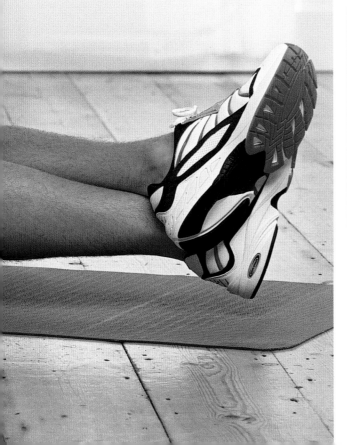

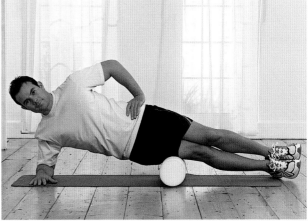

2 Roll over the foam from just below the hip joint down the side of your thigh to the knee. You may find this painful, so do it in moderation intially – the more you do it the less painful it will become. If a 'tender point' is located, stop rolling and rest on the tender point for 20–30 seconds. Repeat on the other side.

quadriceps

1 Lie face down on the floor with one quadriceps (front thigh) on top of the foam roll, supporting your upper body on your forearms. Maintain proper core control, drawing your navel towards your spine to prevent poor posture in your lower back.

2 Roll over the foam from the top of the thigh, just below the pelvic bone, down to the knee, emphasizing the thigh. If a 'tender point' is located, stop rolling and rest on the tender point for 20–30 seconds. Repeat on the other side.

inner thigh

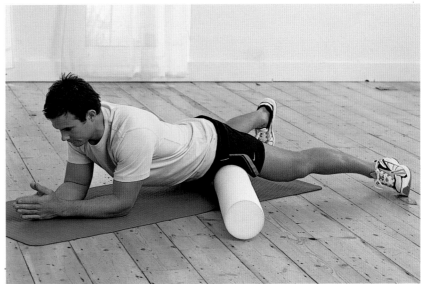

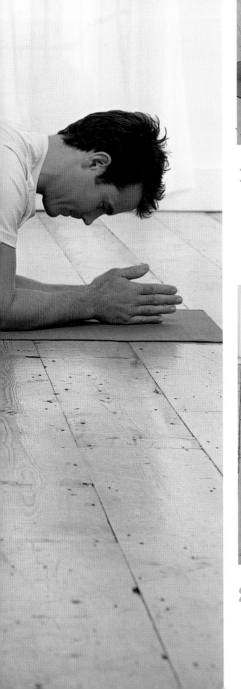

1 Lie face down on the floor with one inner thigh on top of the foam roll, supporting your upper body on your forearms. Turn out the foot of the leg that is being rolled so that its arch is on the floor, thereby exposing the inner thigh. Maintain proper core control, drawing your navel towards your spine to prevent poor posture in your lower back.

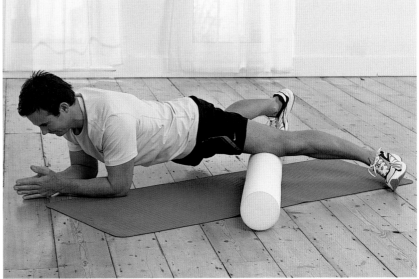

2 Roll over the foam from the top of the inner thigh down to the inner knee. If a 'tender point' is located, stop rolling and rest on the tender point for 20–30 seconds. Repeat on the other side.

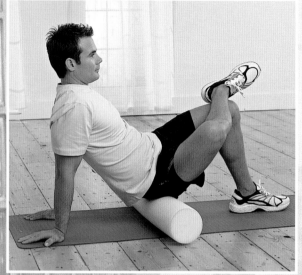

buttocks

Sit on the foam roll, bend your knees and place your feet flat on the floor. Support your body with your hands placed flat on the floor behind you. Cross one foot over the opposite knee to expose the outer side of the buttock of the leg that is raised. Roll this area over the foam, leaning slightly towards that side. If a 'tender point' is located, stop rolling and rest on the tender point for 20–30 seconds. Repeat on the other side.

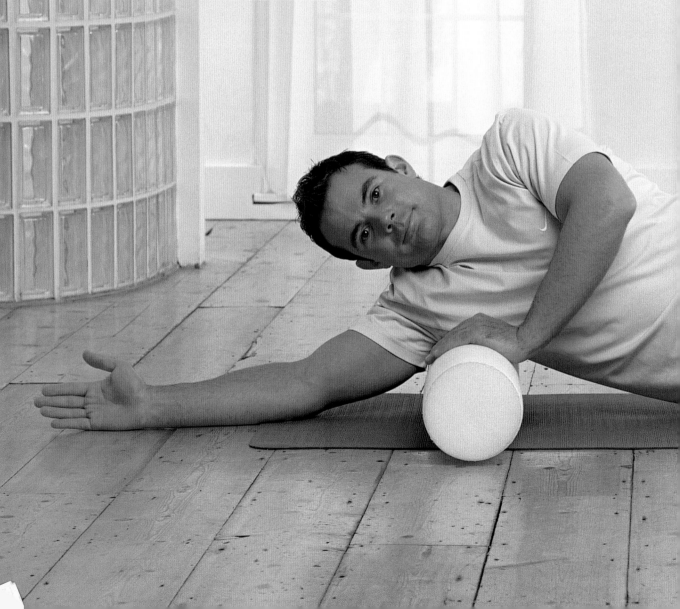

back (lats)

Lie on your side on the floor with one arm outstretched and
the foam roll placed beneath your armpit. Point the thumb
up to prestretch the wing muscle (latissimus dorsi) under
the armpit. Support your body with your free hand and foot
as shown. Movement during this technique is minimal –
explore the muscle by leaning slightly forwards and
backwards on the foam, taking care not to roll down on to
your ribs. If a 'tender point' is located, stop rolling and
rest on the tender point for 20–30 seconds. Repeat on the
other side.

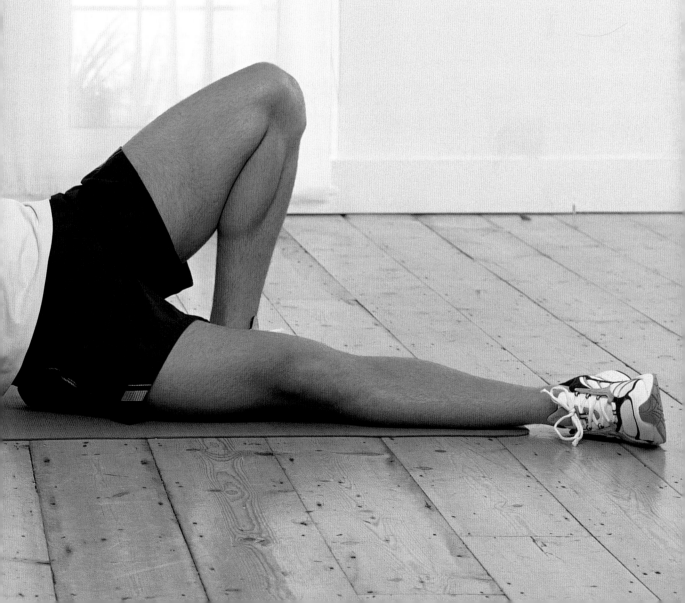

middle back (rhomboids)

1   Lie flat on your back on top of the foam roll with your knees bent and your feet flat on the floor. Position the foam roll across the middle of your back. Raise your hips off the floor and support yourself in a supine bridge position (see pages 80–81). Maintain proper core control, drawing your navel towards your spine to prevent poor posture in your lower back. Stabilize your head position and support your neck using a towel or cushion if necessary. Place your hands across your chest to the opposite shoulders to clear the shoulder blades and expose the musculature.

2   Roll over the foam from your middle back area to just below your neck. If a 'tender point' is located, stop rolling and rest on the tender point for 20–30 seconds.

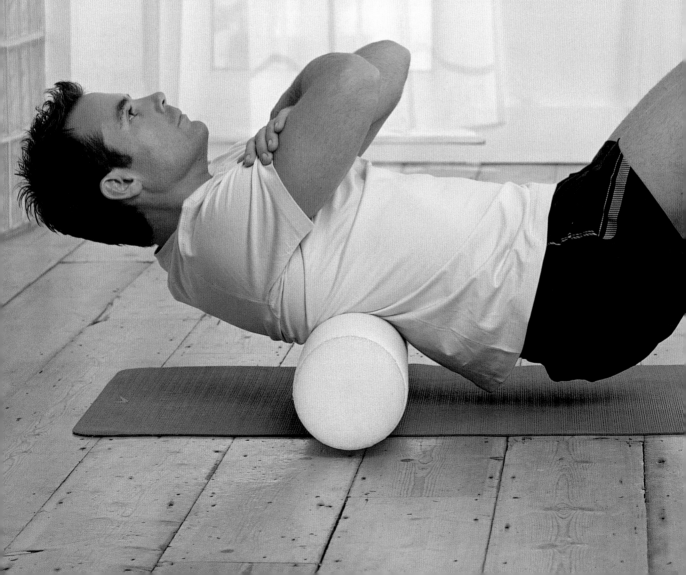

chest

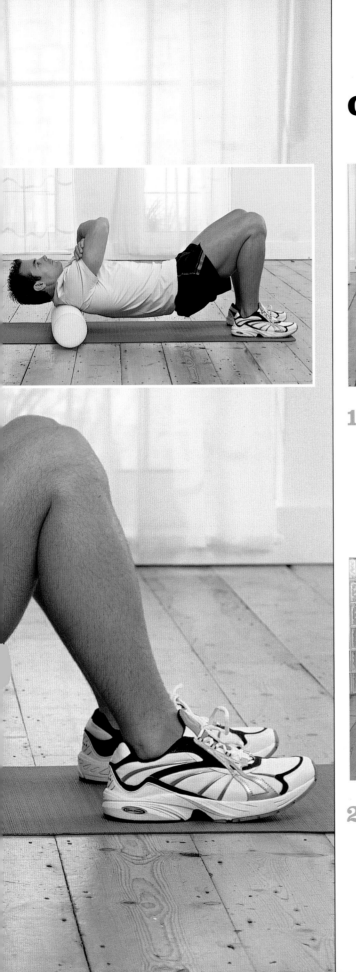

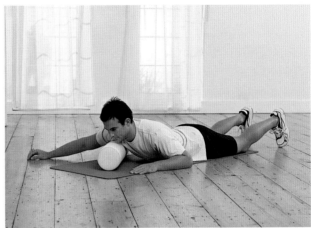

1 Lie face down on the floor with one arm extended and the foam roll at a 45° angle nestled in the crease between the chest and the shoulder. Support your body with the opposite hand and knees. Maintain proper core control, drawing your navel towards your spine to prevent poor posture in your lower back.

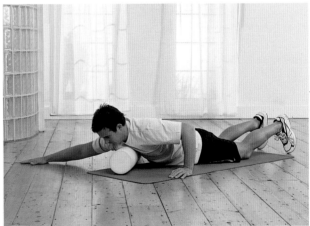

2 Roll your body over the foam on a 45° angle towards the middle of your chest. Be careful not to roll down on to your ribs or your sternum, the bony middle part of your chest. If a 'tender point' is located, stop rolling and rest on the tender point for 20–30 seconds. Repeat on the other side.

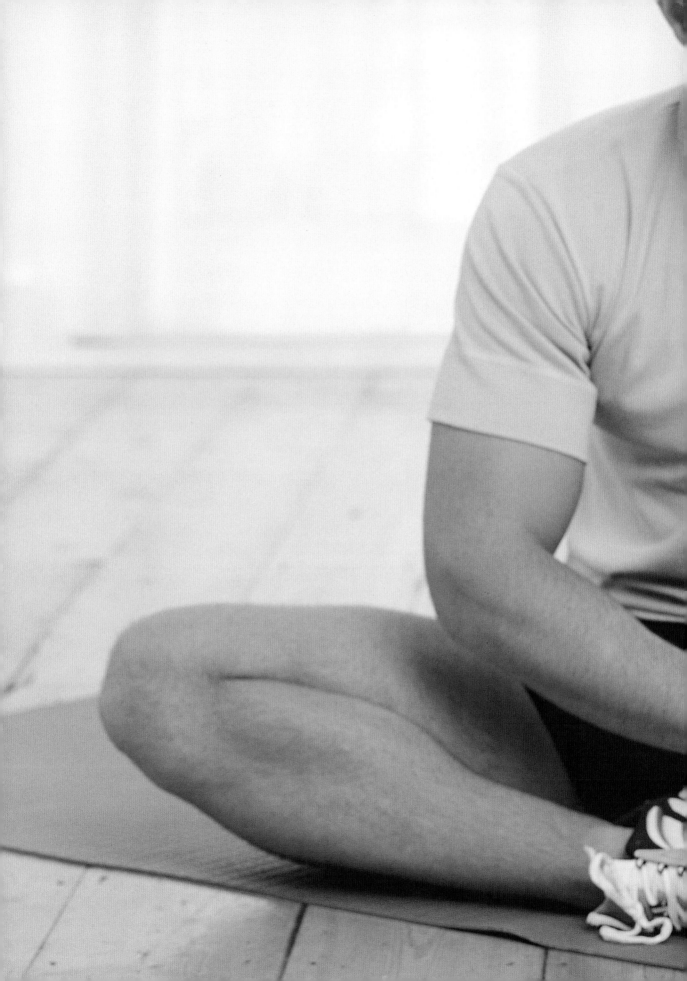

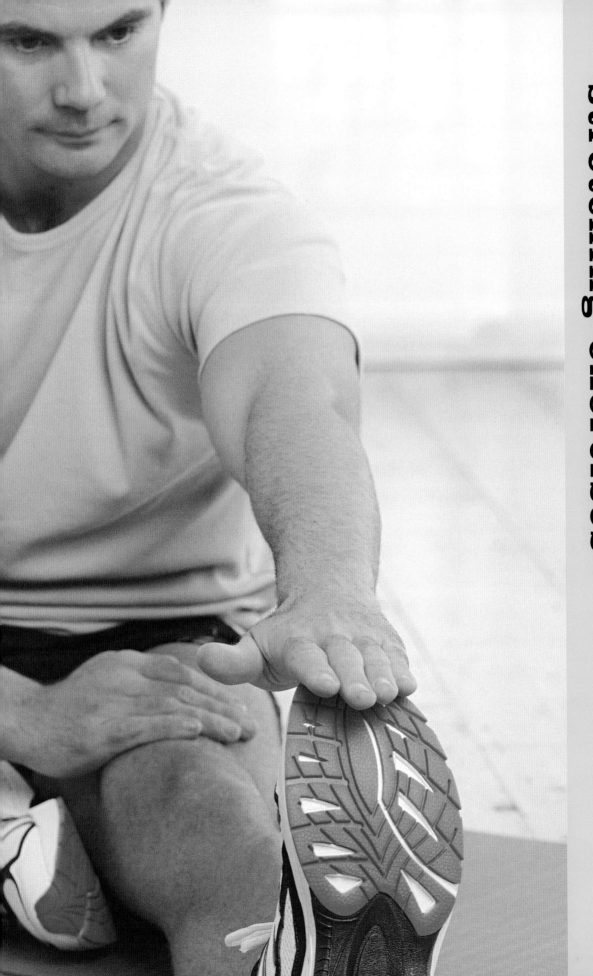

corrective
stretching exercises

Together with SMR foam rolling exercises, static stretches (see pages 57–65) performed regularly and correctly can help improve your flexibility and posture, as well as muscle performance. The exercises should also form a part of every warming up and cooling down session for the body conditioning programme for weeks 1–8. In order for the stretches to make a good impact on your body, make sure you pay particular attention to your form and technique.

Active stretches (see pages 66–75) comprise part of the body conditioning programme for weeks 9–12, by which stage your body should be feeling more flexible thanks to the static stretching exercises from the earlier weeks. Active stretches should be held for 4 seconds and the exercises consist of groups of five stretches on each side. Make sure you follow the correct form and technique so that the active stretches have the maximum effect on your body.

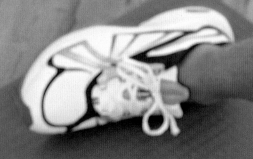
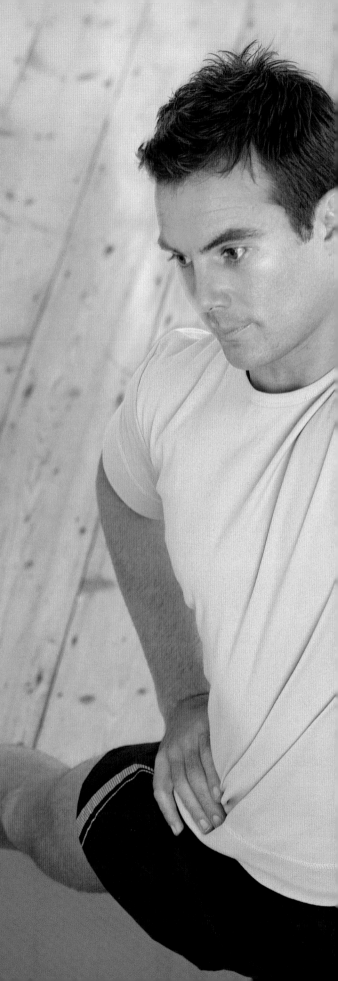

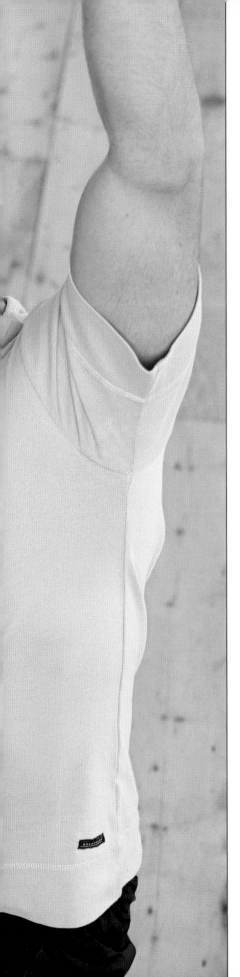

calf stretch

Stand facing a wall and lean towards it. Place your hands on the wall at shoulder height and step forward with one leg to provide support. The foot of your back leg should be flat on the floor pointing straight ahead. Contract your shin muscles and draw your navel towards your spine. Keeping the rear foot flat, bend your rear knee until you feel a slight tension in your calf. Hold the stretch for 20–30 seconds. Do 2–3 reps on each calf.

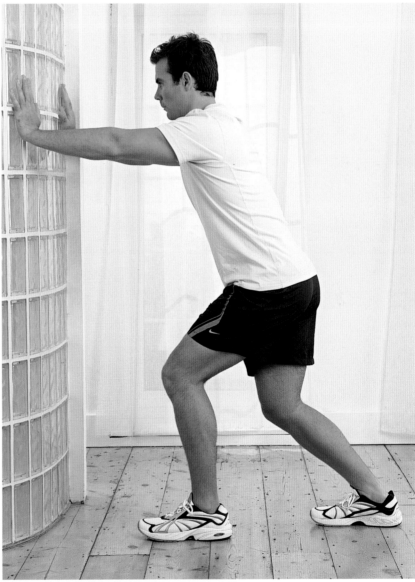

inner thigh and lat stretch

Begin by kneeling on one knee and placing the other leg straight out to the side in line with your body, its foot pointing the way you are facing. Contract your buttocks to help with your alignment and draw your navel towards your spine. Lean your upper body towards the outstretched leg, keeping your body in line with the leg, and reach in the same direction with the opposite arm. Hold the stretch for 20–30 seconds. Do 2–3 reps on each side of your body.

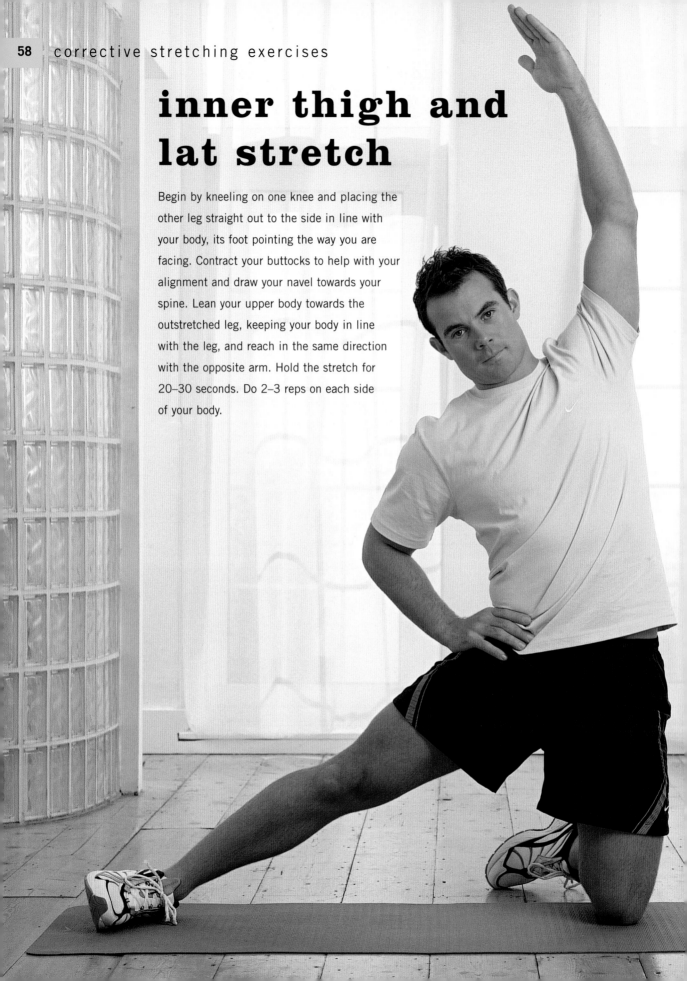

hip and thigh stretch

Lunge down to rest on the floor on one knee, keeping it directly below your hip. Raise the arm and contract the buttock on your kneeling side. Draw your navel towards your spine. Lean into the stretch, keeping your kneeling knee and hip in line with each other. Hold the stretch for 20–30 seconds. Switch sides and repeat.

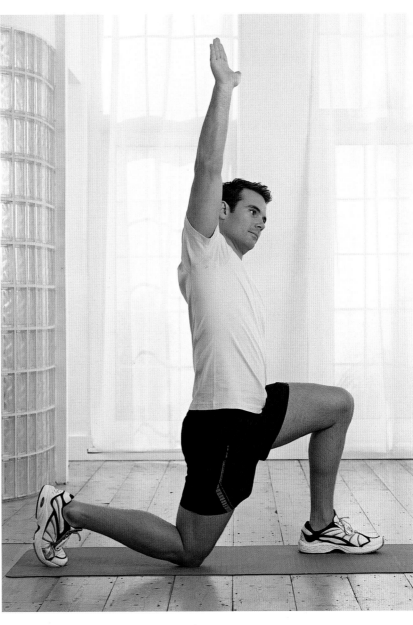

lat stretch

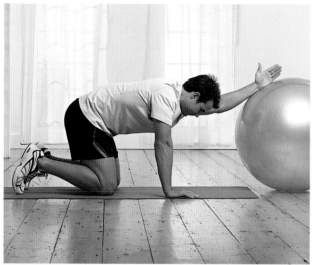

Start by kneeling on all fours. Extend one arm, your palm facing inwards and your thumb pointing to the ceiling, and rest the heel of the palm on a Swiss ball. Push up your lower back. When you feel the first resistance barrier (in other words, the stretch takes hold), hold the stretch for 20–30 seconds. Do 2–3 reps on each side.

You don't have to go to the gym to stretch. You can fit stretching into your day at any time – for example during your lunch break.

chest stretch

Kneel on all fours and draw your navel towards your spine.
Rest one elbow on top of a Swiss ball, ensuring that your
elbow is in line with your shoulder. Contract the shoulder
blades together, keeping them down and back. Exert
downward pressure on the ball through the elbow, rotating
your torso away from the ball. Hold for 20–30 seconds. Do
2–3 reps on each side.

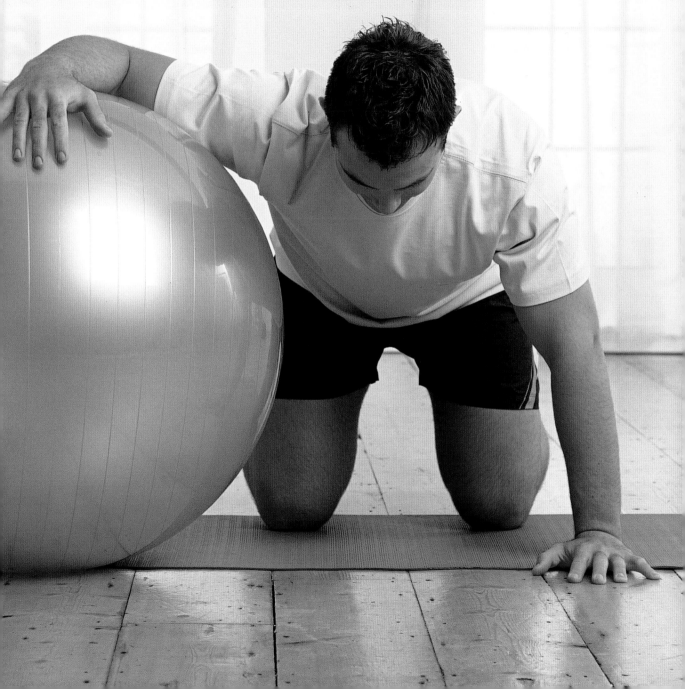

levator scapulae stretch

Sit on a Swiss ball with your feet flat on the floor. Maintain a good posture and draw your navel towards your spine. Place one arm behind your body while keeping your shoulders down and facing back and tucking in your chin. Turn your head to face the shoulder of the other arm. Tilt your head downwards to look down at the floor. Apply gentle pressure to the back of your head with your free hand until you feel the stretch in the back of your neck. Hold for 20–30 seconds. Do 2–3 reps on each side.

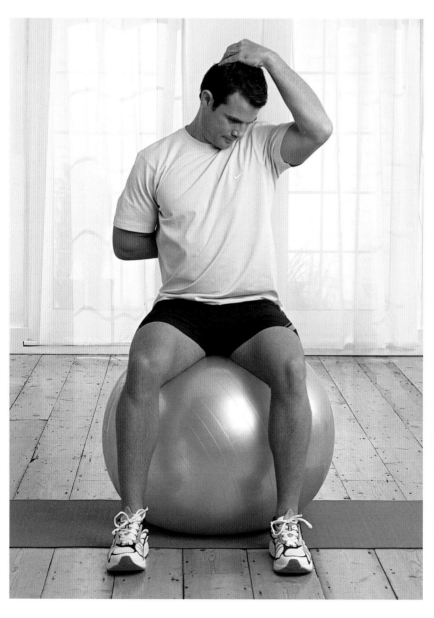
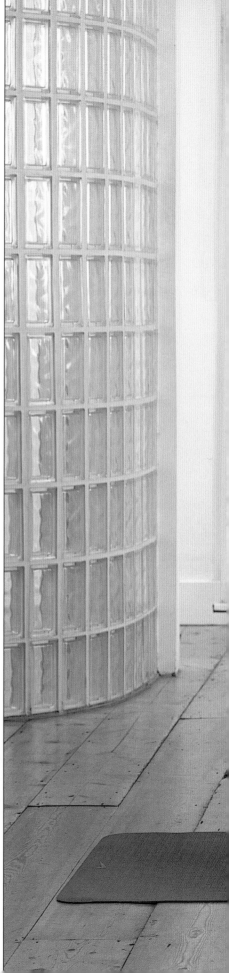

front neck stretch

Sit on a Swiss ball with your feet flat on the floor. Maintain a good posture and draw your navel towards your spine. Place one arm behind your body while keeping your shoulders down and facing back and tucking in your chin. Turn your head to face the shoulder of the other arm. Tilt your head backwards to look up to the ceiling and feel the stretch in the front of your neck. Hold for 20–30 seconds. Do 2–3 reps on each side.

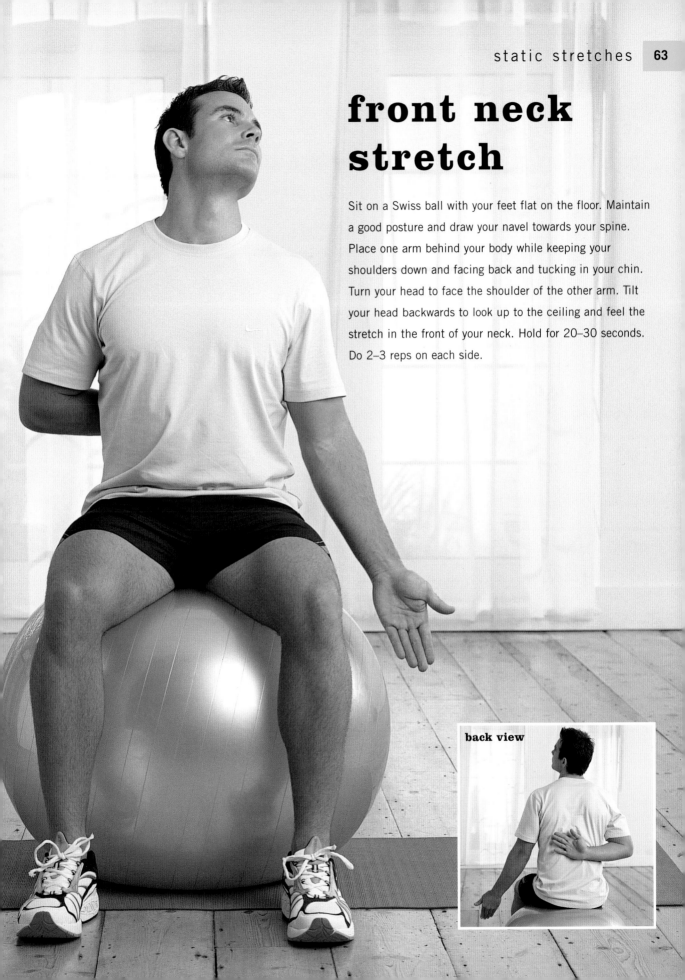

back view

back extension with a swiss ball

Lie flat on your back across a Swiss ball with your knees bent and your feet on the floor. Open up your arms and chest to relax on the ball. Hold the stretch for 30 seconds, making sure that you are not stressing any part of your body – you may find you need a support under your neck.

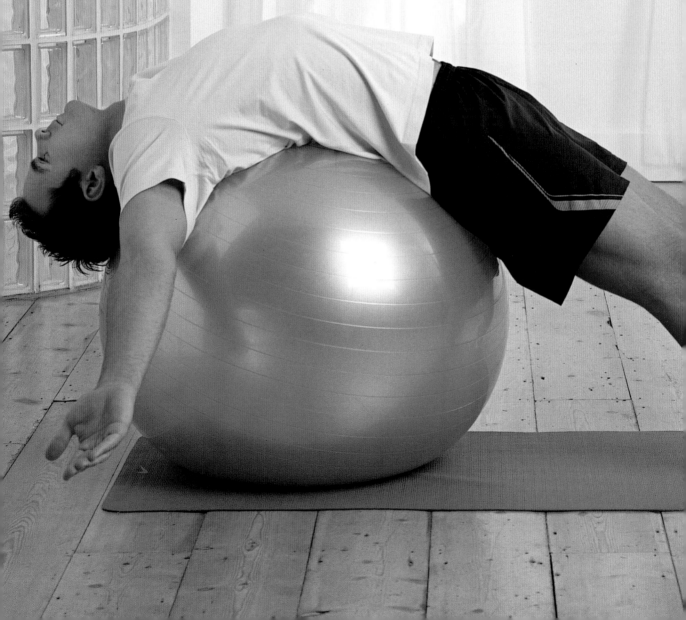

upper trapezius stretch

Sit on a Swiss ball with your feet flat on the floor. Maintain a good posture and draw your navel towards your spine. Place one arm behind your body while keeping your shoulders down and facing back and tucking in your chin. Turn your head to face the shoulder of the other arm. Apply gentle pressure to one side of your head with your free hand until you can feel the stretch in the side of your neck. Hold for 20–30 seconds. Do 2–3 reps on each side.

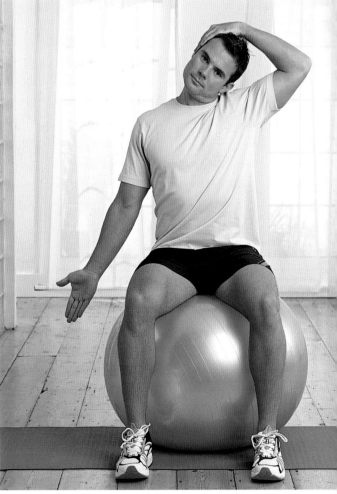

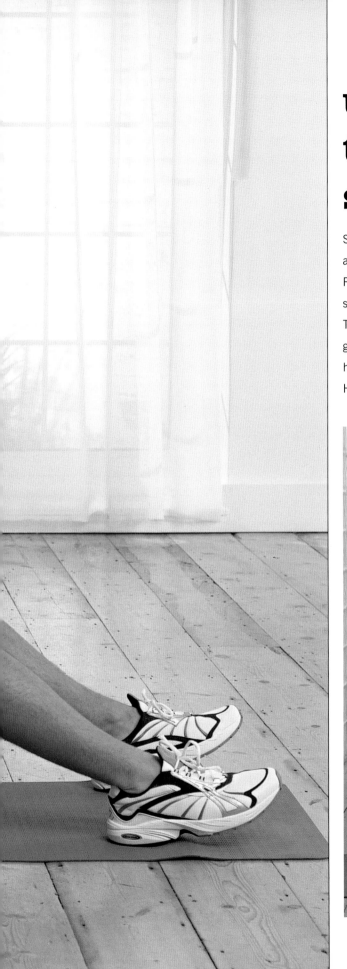

active hip stretch

1 Lunge down to assume a near-kneeling position with one knee just above floor level, the other leg bent at a 90° angle in front of you. Draw your navel towards your spine and squeeze your buttocks while tucking your pelvis under. Slowly, move your body forward until you feel tension in the front of the hip of the rear leg.

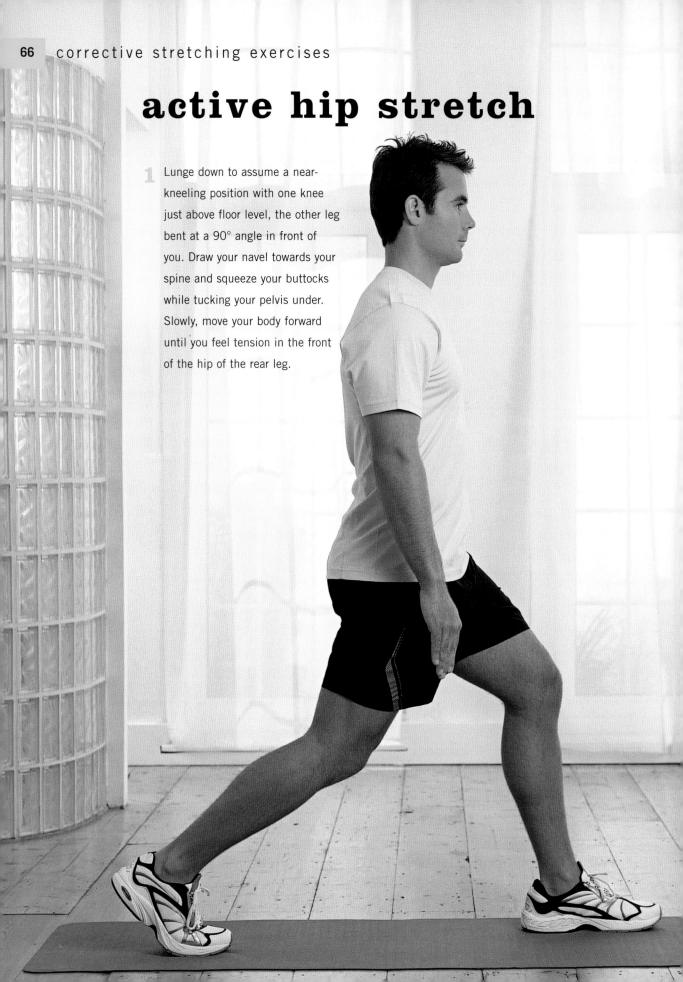

active calf stretch

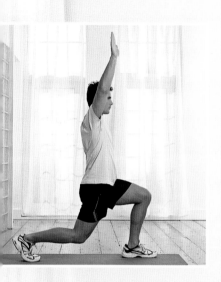

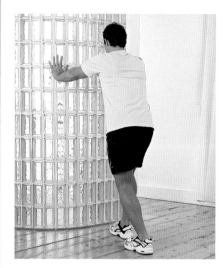

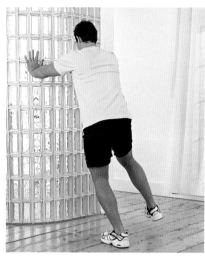

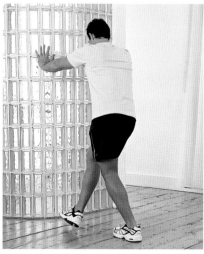

2 Raise the arm on the same side as the hip being stretched and lean your upper body sideways towards the opposite side, while maintaining a stable pelvis. Move in and out of this stretch position in a controlled manner for 4 seconds each side. Do 5 reps on each leg.

1 Stand facing a wall and lean towards it. Place your hands on the wall at shoulder height and step forward with one leg to provide support.

2 Keep your back foot flat on the floor and make sure the knee of this leg is in line with your second and third toes. Draw your navel towards your spine. Flex the knee of the front leg and lift it off the floor. Slowly move through your hips, controlling the movement of the front leg from side to side so as to stretch the calf muscle of the rear leg.

3 Move in and out of the stretch position for 4 seconds on each side. Do 5 reps on each leg.

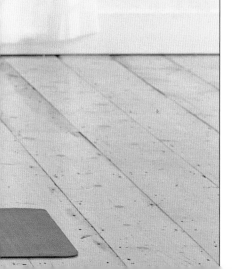

active inner thigh stretch

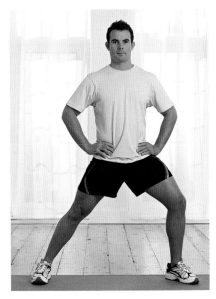

1 Stand with your legs more than shoulder width apart and your hands on your hips. Lean to one side, with your supporting leg pointing 45° away from your body and you other leg pointing straight ahead.

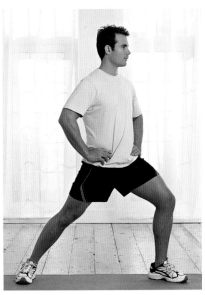

2 Turn your hips so your upper body faces to one side and bend this foremost leg. Draw your navel towards your spine, tuck your pelvis under and lean into the stretch maintaining good posture. When you have felt the tension in your inside leg, rotate your hips back towards the supporting leg. Move in and out of this stretch position in a controlled manner for 4 seconds each side. Do 5 reps on each leg.

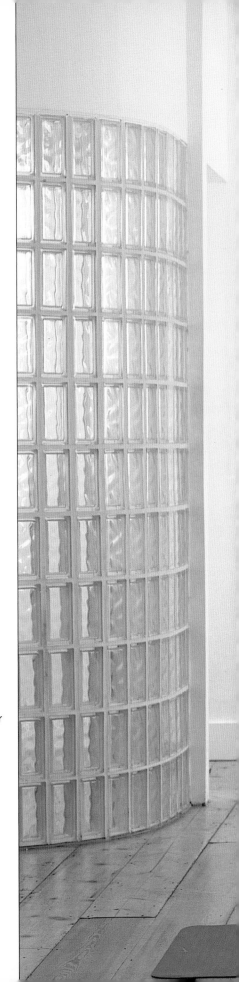

active hip and lat stretch

1 Stand with one leg behind the other, your feet facing forward. Extend the arm belonging to the same side of your body as the rear leg towards the ceiling.

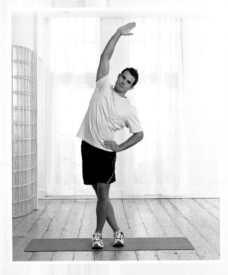

2 Draw your navel towards your spine and squeeze your buttocks while tilting your body to the side and reaching up and across with the extended arm. Control the movement until you feel the stretch in your hip and lats, while maintaining a neutral pelvis. Hold for 4 seconds. Do 5 reps on each side.

active lat stretch

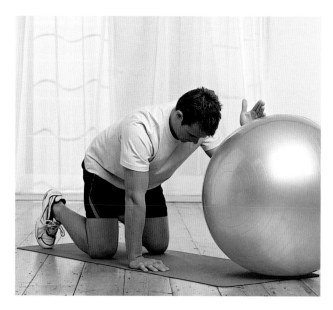

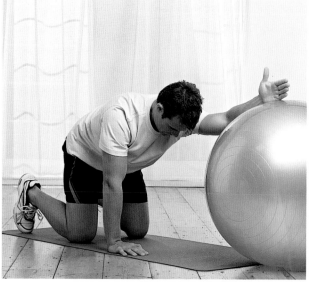

1 Kneel on all fours in front of a Swiss ball. Extend one arm, your palm facing inwards and your thumb pointing to the ceiling, and rest the heel of the palm on the ball.

2 Draw your navel towards your spine. Maintaining a neutral pelvis, roll the ball away from you until you can feel a comfortable stretch underneath your arm.

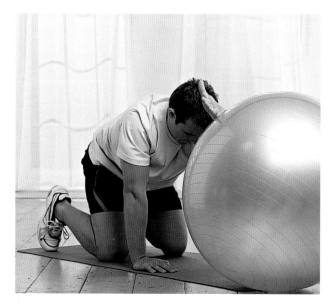

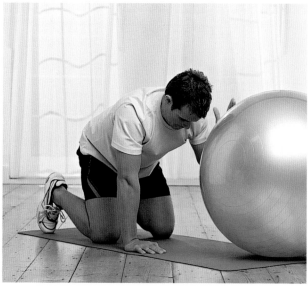

4 Next roll the ball in the same fashion at an angle across your body.

5 Hold for 4 seconds before returning to your starting position.

chest stretch

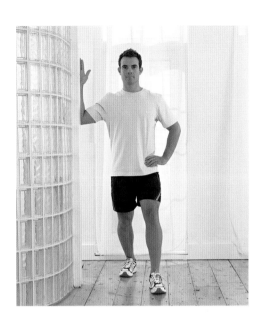

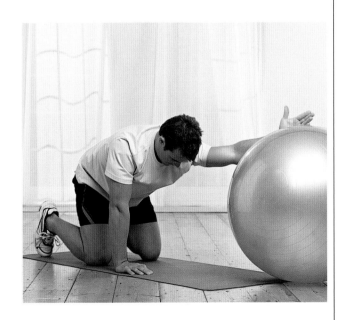

3 Hold for 4 seconds then return to your starting position.

1 Stand directly in front of a wall or heavy object. Lift one arm to shoulder height, flex to form a 90° angle at the elbow and place your hand against the wall.

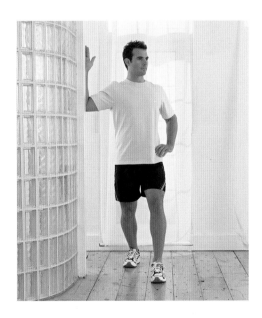

6 Finally, roll the ball to the side away from you and hold for 4 seconds before returning to your starting position again. Do 5 reps on each arm.

2 Squeeze your shoulder blades together. Slowly rotate your trunk away from the stationary arm until you can feel a slight stretch in your chest and the front of your shoulders. Hold for 4 seconds. Do 5 reps on each side.

active neck stretch

Sit on a Swiss ball with your feet flat on the floor and your arms tucked behind your back, your knuckles against your body. Maintain a good posture and draw your navel towards your spine.

warm-up squats

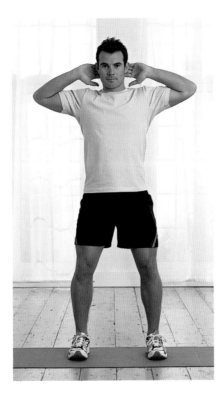

1 Stand tall with a good posture, holding your hands behind your head. Draw your navel towards your spine.

2 Tuck in your chin and draw your left ear to your left shoulder. Progress by rotating your head so that you face the ceiling. Hold for 4 seconds, all the time keeping your shoulders down and facing back. Switch direction and repeat the move. Do 5 reps on each side.

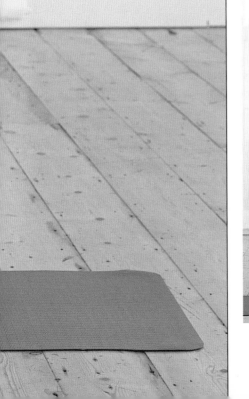

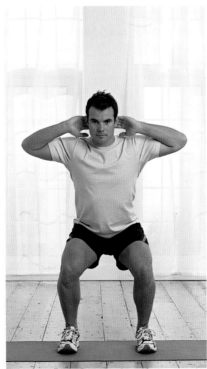

2 Lower yourself to a squat position in a controlled manner, pushing your bottom and hips behind you as though about to sit down. Keep your knees and toes in alignment and hold for 4 seconds. Return to a standing position, coming up on to your toes. Do 5 reps.

IT band squats

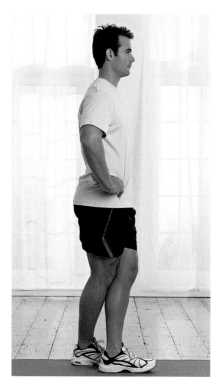

1 Stand with one leg behind the other, your feet facing forward and your hands on your hips. Draw your navel towards your spine.

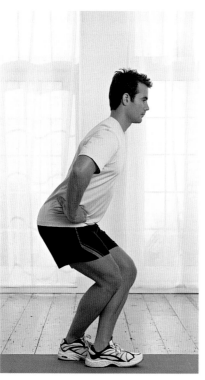

2 Lower yourself to a squat position in a controlled manner, pushing your bottom and hips behind you as though about to sit down, and keeping your feet facing forward. Hold for 4 seconds before returning to your starting position. Switch legs and repeat. Do 5 reps on each leg.

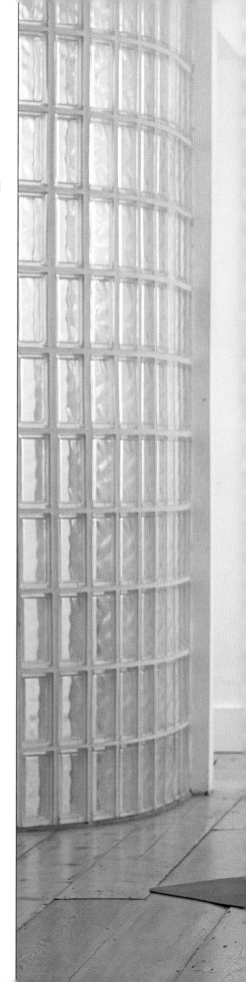

lunge with rotation

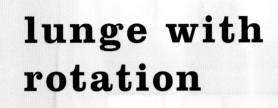

1 Stand tall with a good posture, your arms extended in front of you at chest height and your palms together. Draw your navel towards your spine. Maintaining total body alignment, step forward and lower yourself slowly by flexing your hips, knees and ankles.

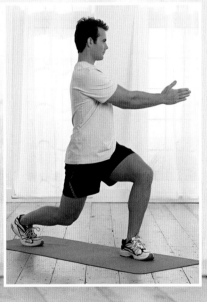

Slowly rotate your spine to the side, towards the front leg, lowering yourself into a lunge position, and hold for 4 seconds. Use your hip and thigh muscles to push yourself back to your starting position. Switch legs and repeat. Do 5 reps on each leg.

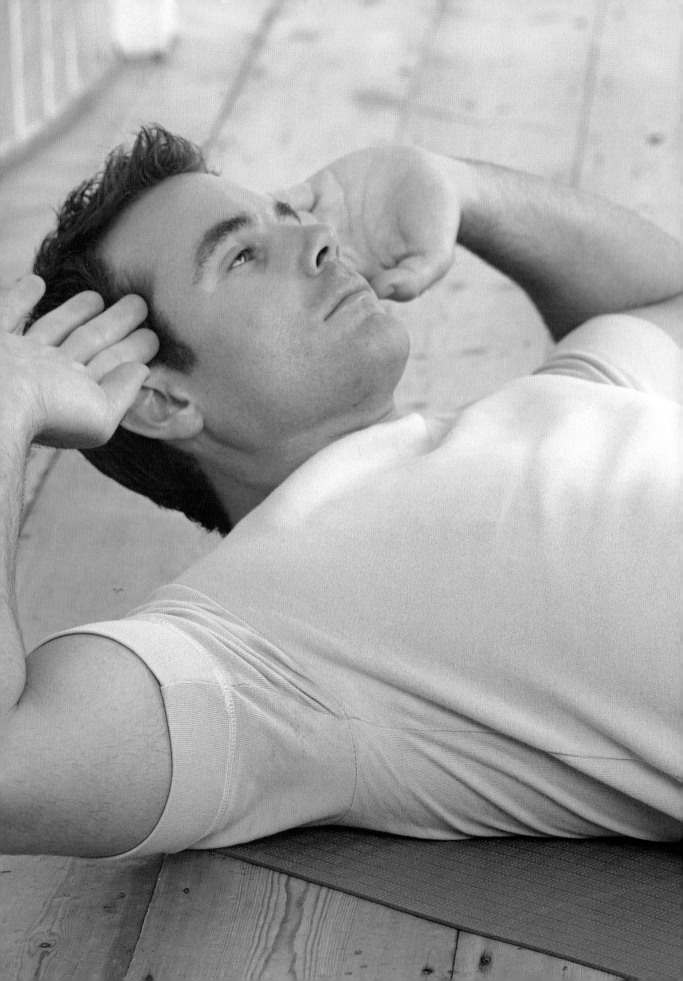

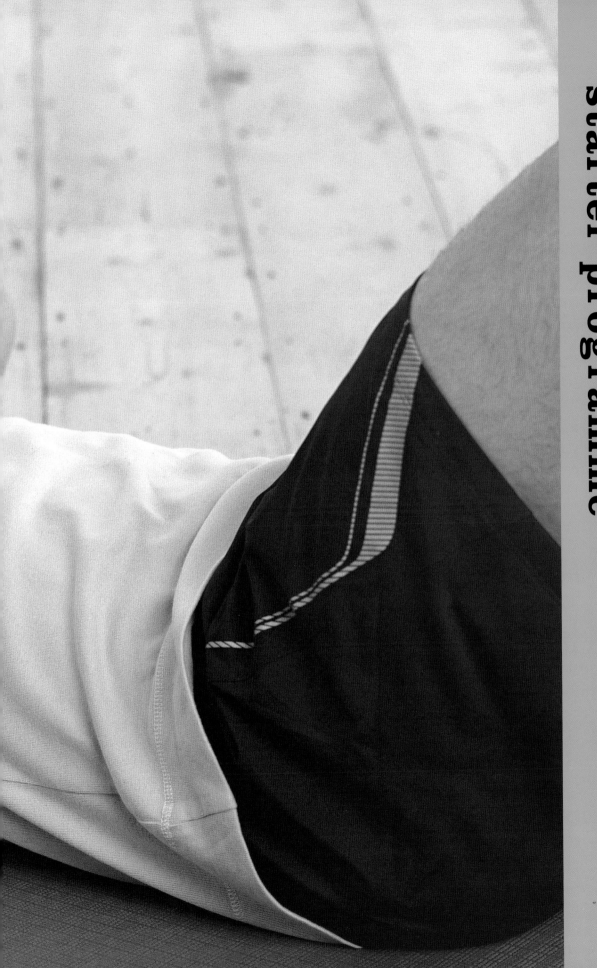

weeks 1–4
starter programme

starter programme

The programme for the initial four weeks is intended to get someone who is out of condition back into exercise or to reteach someone who has already been training but who has poor postural habits. The starter programme introduces a corrective stretching routine, emphasizing the use of your core, balance and reaction time (abilities that are all reduced in an out-of-condition person), with the aims of getting your body systems to work together as a unit and to build a strong base of support that can be improved upon. The CV training can be done at the end of the body conditioning exercises or on alternate days on its own with a full warm-up and cool-down.

The starter programme should take you 35–45 minutes, in addition to the warm-up and cool-down and any CV work, and you should do it twice a week.

weeks 1–4 programme order

■ warm-up (15 minutes)

• SMR foam rolling (see pages 44–53)
• Corrective stretching (see 'Static stretches', pages 56–65)
• 5-minute moderate CV exercise (see page 24)

■ body conditioning exercises

• Floor supine bridge (see pages 80–81)
• Floor cobra (see page 81)
• Drawing-in manoeuvre (see page 82)
• Single-leg balance (see page 83)
• Jump (optional) (see pages 84–85)
• Squat bicep curl (see page 86)
• Chest press on foam roll (see pages 86–87)
• Ball row with resistance (see page 89)
• Standing scaption (see pages 88–89)
• Squat (see page 90)
• Lunge (see pages 90–91)

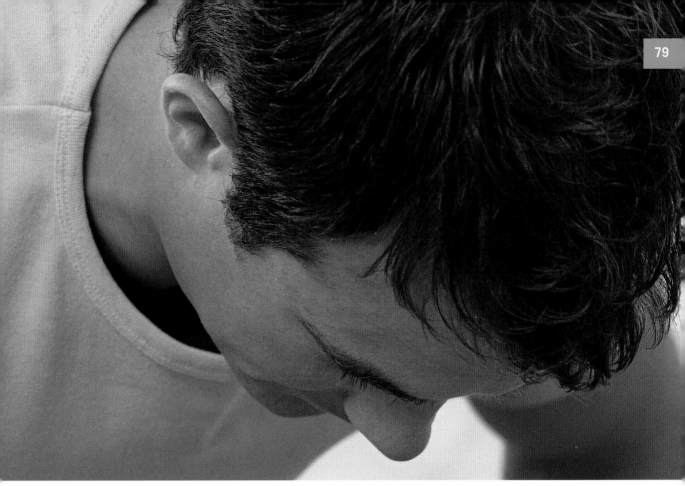

■ cv training

Intensity 50–65 per cent of your maximum heart rate

Duration 30 minutes

Frequency two times a week – after the body conditioning exercises, or on alternate days to the exercises

■ cool-down (15 minutes)

• 5-minute moderate CV exercise (see page 24)

• SMR foam rolling (see pages 44–53)

• Corrective stretching (see 'Static stretches', pages 56–65)

reps	15
sets	1
tempo	4-2-2
benefits	works the buttocks and core

floor supine bridge

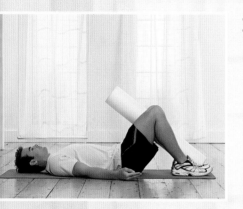

1 Begin by lying flat on your back on the floor with your knees bent, your feet flat, your toes pointing straight ahead and your arms by your sides. Activate your core by drawing your navel towards your spine and squeezing your buttocks. Squeezing a foam roll between your knees helps keep your hips flat and activate your core.

2 With activated core and squeezed buttocks, lift your hips off the floor to form a straight line between your knees and shoulders. Hold then slowly return to your starting position. Touch the floor momentarily then repeat.

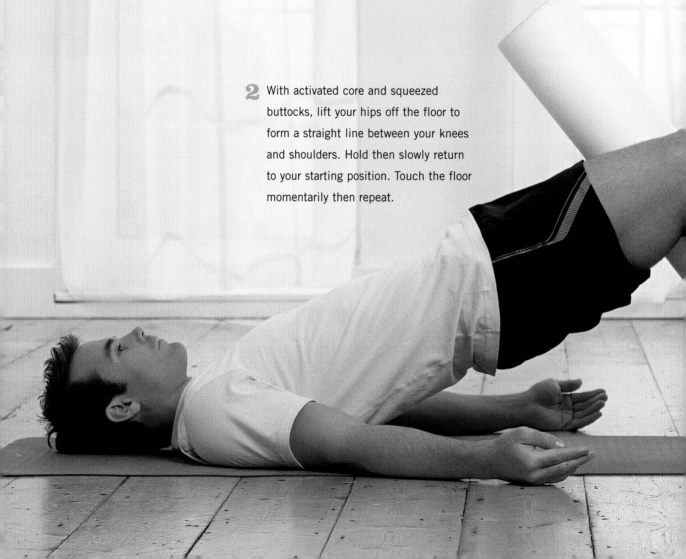

reps   15
sets   1
tempo   4-2-2
benefits   strengthens the core,
and works the buttocks,
middle and lower back

floor cobra

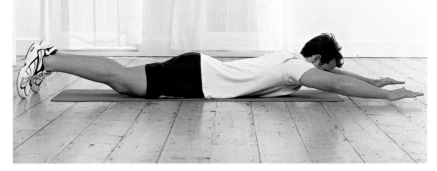

1 Lie face down on the floor with your arms extended beyond your head and your palms flat on the floor. Activate your core by drawing your navel towards your spine and squeezing your buttocks.

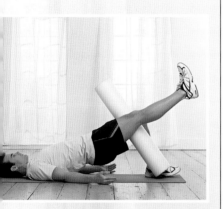

progression Increase the intensity of the exercise by keeping one leg raised.

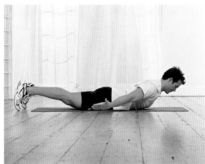

2 Lift your chest off the floor, bring your arms back towards your hips, rotating your thumbs towards the ceiling. Pause momentarily at the top of the lift then return to your starting position and repeat.

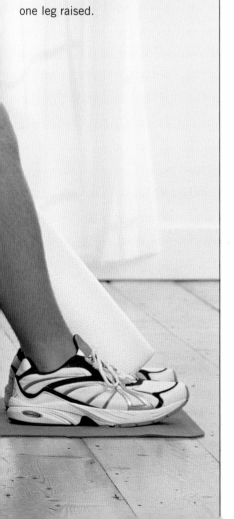

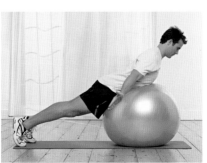

progression Perform the same exercise while resting on a Swiss ball.

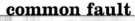
common fault

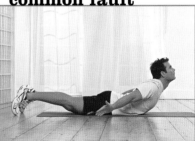

Take care not to arch your back when you lift your chest off the floor.

reps	15
sets	1
tempo	4-2-2
benefits	increases the ability to activate the core to help with stability

drawing-in

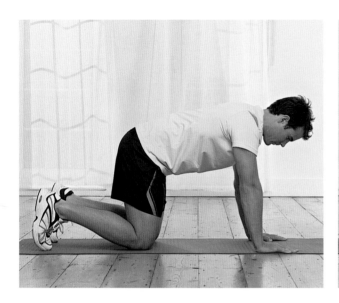

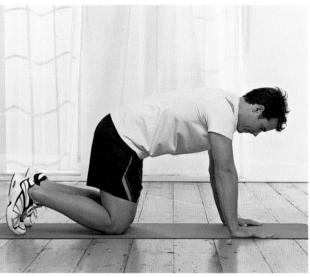

1 Kneel on all fours, ensuring you have a neutral spine from head to tail bone.

2 Draw your lower abdomen up and in while breathing naturally. The lower abdomen should elevate before the upper. Maintain a neutral spinal position – there should be no movement from the spine while drawing inwards. Hold for 4 seconds and release then repeat.

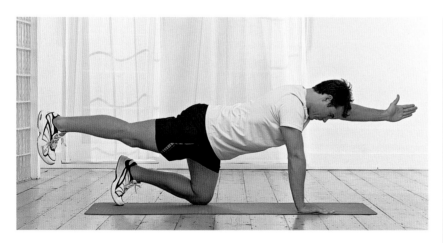

progression Perform the same exercise, with one arm and the opposite leg extended so that you are balancing on just one hand and one knee.

common fault

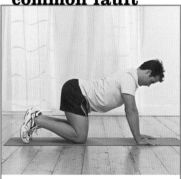

Take care not to tilt your pelvis forwards or backwards. Keep neutral alignment.

reps	15
sets	1
tempo	4-2-2
benefits	improves balance and mind–muscle connection

single-leg balance

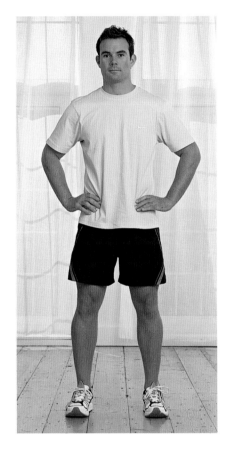

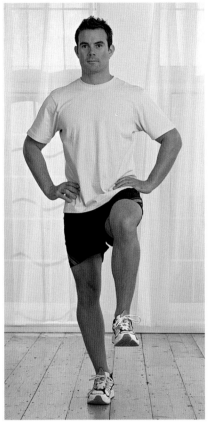

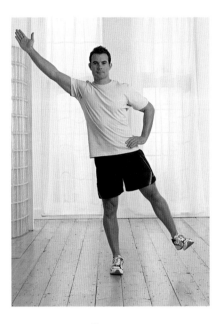

progression Extend your free leg to the side and extend the opposite arm.

1 Stand tall with your legs shoulder width apart and your hands on your hips. Activate your core by drawing your navel towards your spine. Stabilize your hips by squeezing your buttocks, maintain a neutral spine position and keep your hips level.

2 Slowly lift one leg off the floor and hold the position, standing on the remaining leg with its foot pointing straight ahead and knee slightly flexed while maintaining a stable position in line with your second and third toes. Maintain a good posture – your shoulders should be down and facing back, the angle of your spine neutral. Return to your starting position and repeat.

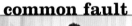

common fault

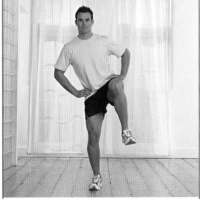

Don't allow your hips drop or your body to rotate out of alignment.

reps 6
sets 1
tempo land and hold for 3 seconds
benefits improves deceleration, stabilization and neuromuscular control

jump

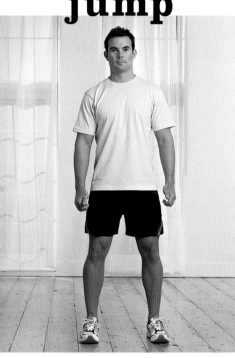

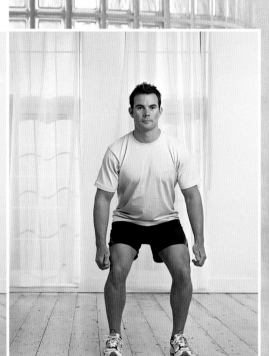

1 Stand with your legs shoulder width apart, your knees in line with your second and third toes and your arms held ready to help you with this movement.

2 Squat down slightly then jump explosively to one side. Land on your toes, then your heels. Repeat on the other side.

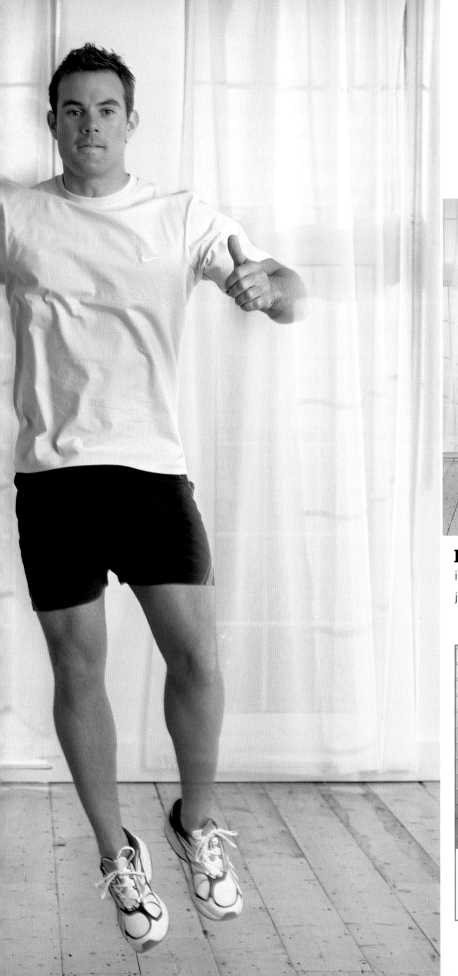

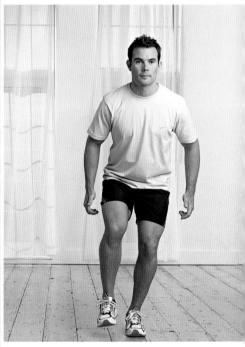

progression Increase the intensity by standing and jumping on just one leg, then the other.

common fault

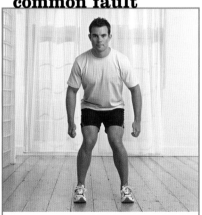

Don't let your hips, knees and toes fall out of alignment.

reps	12
sets	1
tempo	3-2-1
benefits	increases core stabilization, integrating the core and upper and lower body

squat bicep curl

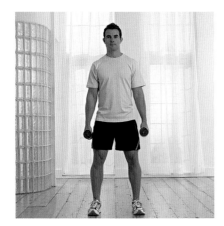

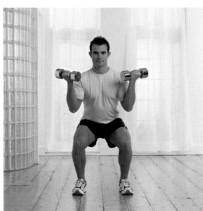

1 Stand with your legs shoulder width apart, your arms down by your sides with a dumbbell in each hand, palms facing inwards. Activate your core by drawing your navel towards your spine. Stabilize yourself and keep your hips level by squeezing your buttocks. Maintain a neutral spine position.

2 Ensuring your posture is good – keeping your shoulders down and facing back, and your spine neutral – lower yourself slightly, pushing your bottom and hips behind you as though about to sit down. At the same time perform a bicep curl by flexing your elbows and bringing the dumbbells up towards your shoulders. Keeping your upper arms still and your palms facing forward, slowly return to your starting position then repeat.

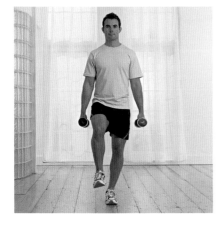

progression Perform the exercise while standing on just one leg, then the other.

reps	12
sets	1
tempo	3-2-1
benefits	increases strength in the chest and secondary core/buttocks

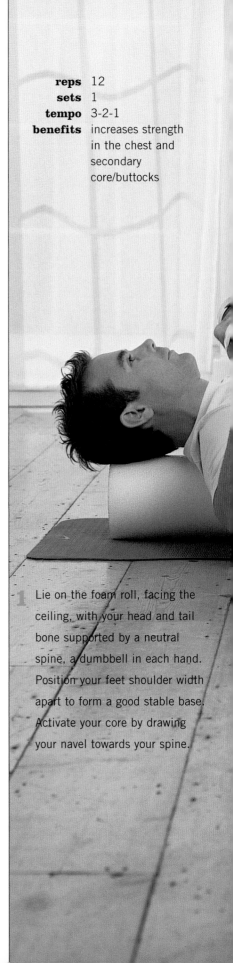

1 Lie on the foam roll, facing the ceiling, with your head and tail bone supported by a neutral spine, a dumbbell in each hand. Position your feet shoulder width apart to form a good stable base. Activate your core by drawing your navel towards your spine.

chest press on foam roll

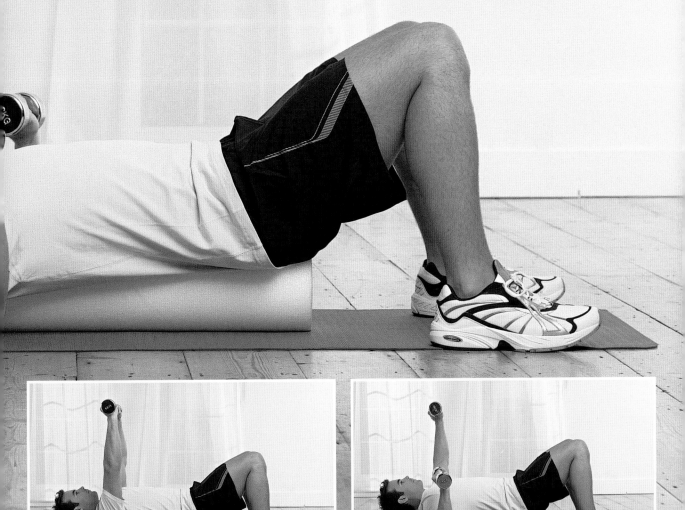

Begin with the weights on your chest. Slowly push the dumbbells as far as you can towards the ceiling while exhaling. When at the top bring the dumbbells back down to your chest while inhaling, then repeat the movement.

progression Raise a single arm at a time.

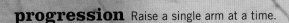

reps   12
sets   1
tempo   3-2-1
benefits   strengthens the rotator cuff group of muscles (the shoulder girdle)

standing scaption

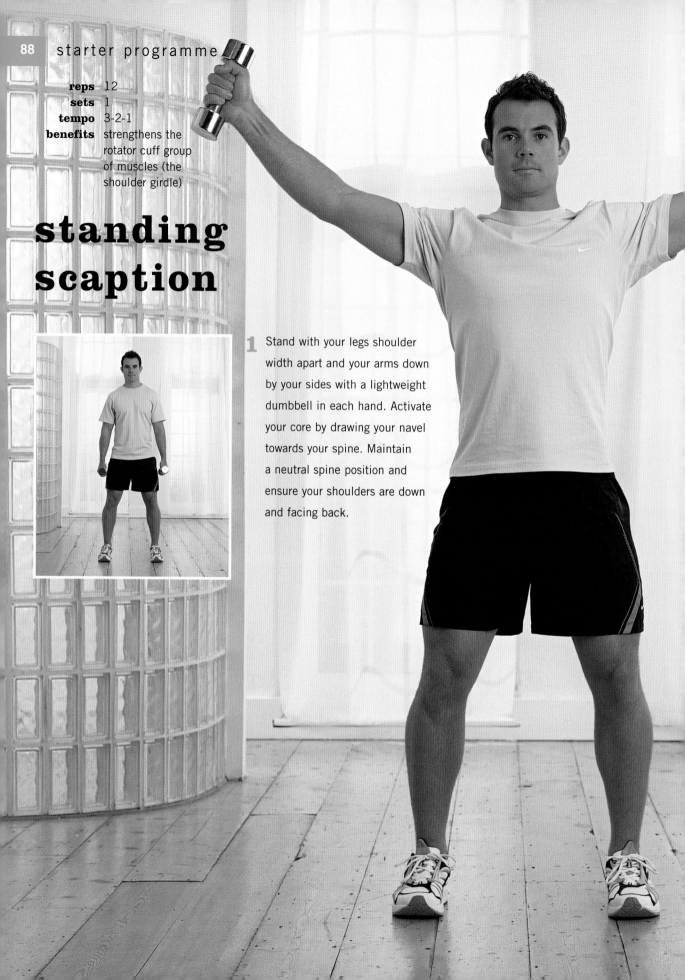

1 Stand with your legs shoulder width apart and your arms down by your sides with a lightweight dumbbell in each hand. Activate your core by drawing your navel towards your spine. Maintain a neutral spine position and ensure your shoulders are down and facing back.

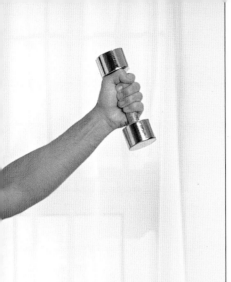

reps	12
sets	1
tempo	3-2-1
benefits	strengthens the core, buttocks, shoulders and back

ball row with resistance

2 Raising your arms from your shoulder joints, turn both arms out until your chest is open. Then return to your starting position and repeat.

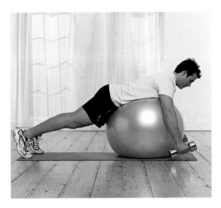

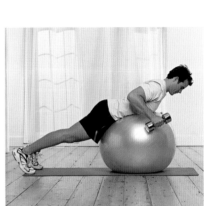

1 Lay face down across a Swiss ball, with the ball beneath the middle of your chest. Holding a dumbbell in each hand, extend your arms out in front of you. Ensure your legs are straight behind you, and your core is activated with your navel drawn towards your spine.

2 Squeeze your buttocks and draw your shoulder blades back and downwards, bringing your elbows in close to the side of your body. Your chin should be tucked in as you lift your torso off the Swiss ball. Return to your starting position then repeat.

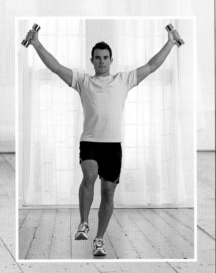

progression Perform the exercise standing on just one leg.

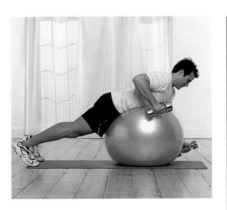

progression Perform the exercise bringing just one arm at a time back into your body.

common fault

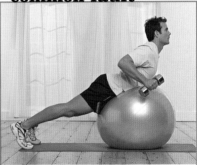

Take care not to arch your back when you lift your chest off the Swiss ball.

reps	12
sets	1
tempo	3-2-1
benefits	improves total body stability and strength, with emphasis on the lower body

squat

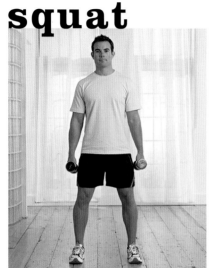

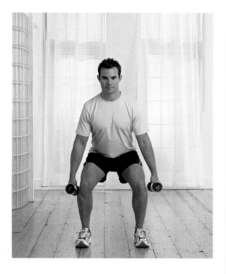

1 Stand with your legs shoulder width apart or wider, your knees in line with your second or third toes. Hold your arms down by your sides with a dumbbell in each hand, ensuring your shoulders are down and facing back.

2 Draw your navel towards your spine. Keeping your spine neutral, lower yourself slowly into a squat position by bending at the knees and hips, pushing your bottom and hips behind you as though about to sit down. Return to your starting position and repeat. Perform the downward reps slowly and concentrate on the descent and the finish position. Descend as far as you can while still maintaining good control. Partial squats should progress to full squats as you improve.

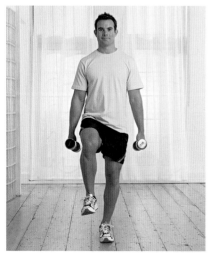

progression Perform the exercise while standing on just one leg, then the other.

lunge

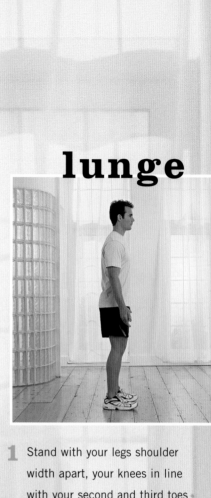

1 Stand with your legs shoulder width apart, your knees in line with your second and third toes and your arms down by your sides. Draw your navel towards your spine.

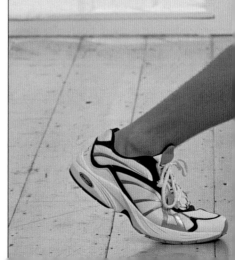

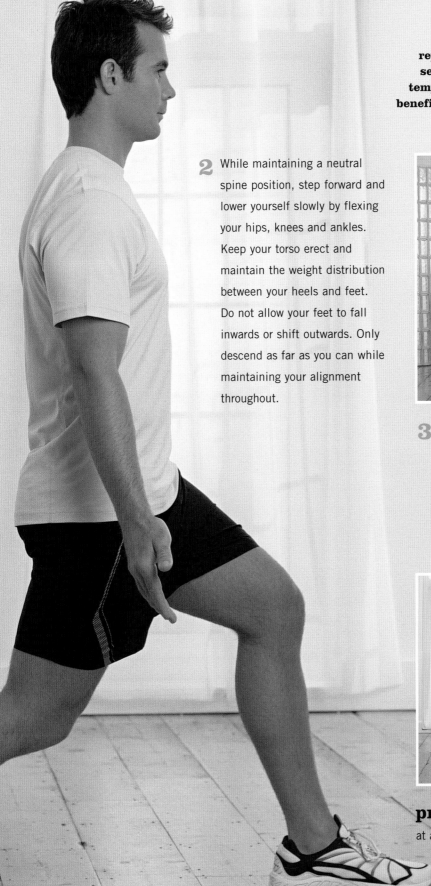

reps 12
sets 1
tempo 3-2-1
benefits strengthens the legs and improves total body stability

2 While maintaining a neutral spine position, step forward and lower yourself slowly by flexing your hips, knees and ankles. Keep your torso erect and maintain the weight distribution between your heels and feet. Do not allow your feet to fall inwards or shift outwards. Only descend as far as you can while maintaining your alignment throughout.

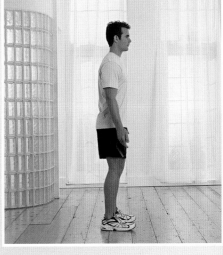

3 Return slowly to your starting position then repeat. Perform the downwards reps slowly, concentrating on the descent and the alignment of your body. Do 2 sets of 12 reps on each leg.

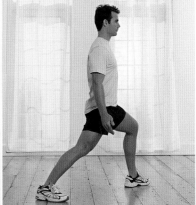

progression Lunge forwards at a 45° angle.

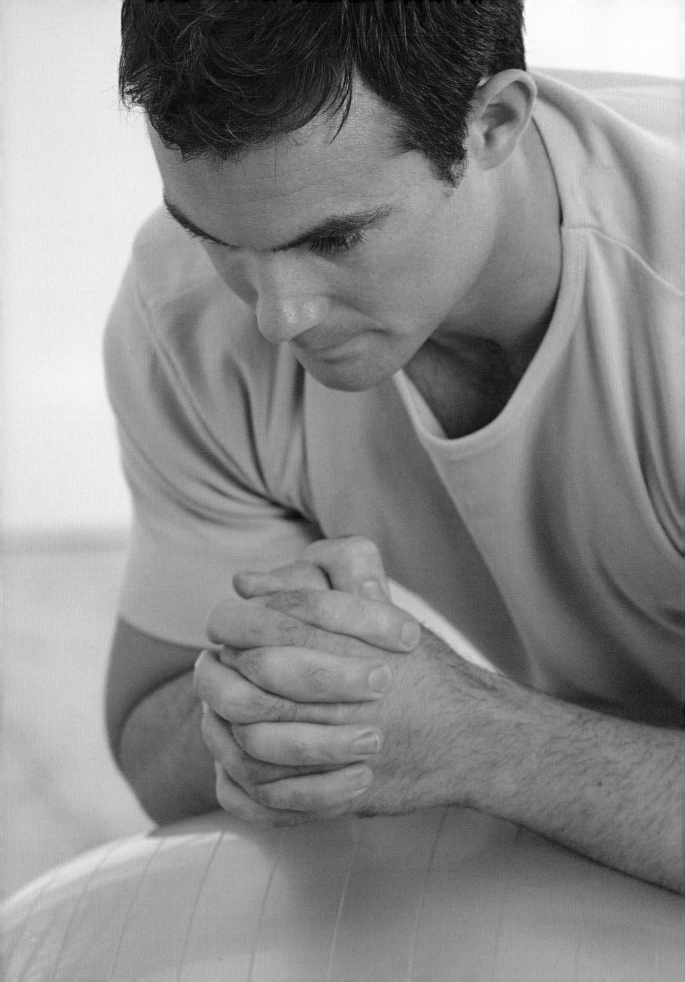

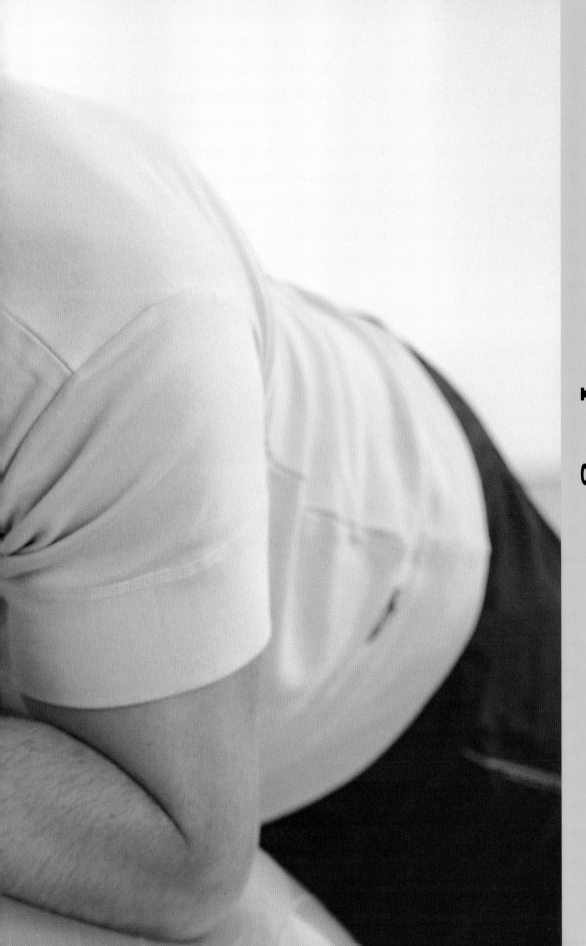

weeks 5-8
intermediate programme

intermediate programme

The intermediate phase of the body conditioning programme builds on the stability and improved muscular function gained from the initial four weeks of training. Developing better movement patterns, skills and adaptations to exercise is the purpose of weeks 5–8, as well as enhancing your endurance, cultivating the benefits of improved functional flexibility and progressing towards an increased level of intensity and challenges with a reduced risk of injury. Once again, the CV training can be done at the end of the body conditioning exercises or on its own on another day with

a full warm-up and cool-down. Do CV training 1 once a week and CV training 2 (interval training) once a week, giving you a total of two CV workouts per week.

The intermediate programme should take you 35–45 minutes, in addition to the warm-up and cool-down and any CV work, and you should do it three times a week.

weeks 5–8 programme order

■ warm-up (15 minutes)

- SMR foam rolling (see pages 44–53)
- Corrective stretching (see 'Static stretches', pages 56–65)
- 5-minute moderate CV exercise (see page 24)

■ body conditioning exercises

- Prone isolation abs (see page 96)
- Ball crunch (see pages 96–97)
- Multi-direction hop (see pages 98–99)
- Balance (see page 99)
- Squat single-leg balance (see pages 100–101)
- Swiss ball T-row (see pages 102–103)
- Swiss ball chest press (see page 103)
- Swiss ball military press (see page 104)
- Standing scaption (see page 105)
- Lunge (see pages 106–107)

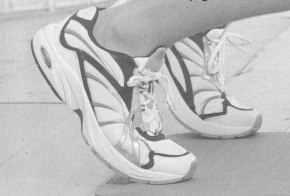

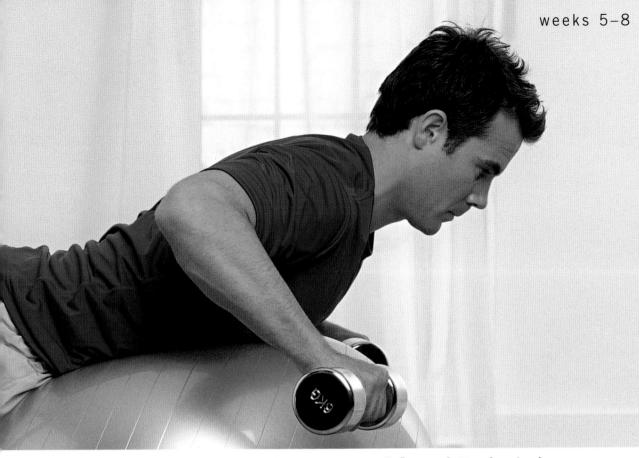

▣ cv training 1 or 2

▣ cv training 1

Intensity 50–65 per cent of your maximum heart rate

Duration 45 minutes

Frequency once a week – after the body conditioning exercises or on other days

▣ cv training 2

Intensity Interval training, i.e. 65 per cent of your maximum heart rate for 1 minute/85 per cent of your maximum heart rate for 1 minute, consecutively

Duration 30 minutes

Frequency once a week – after the body conditioning exercises or on another day

▣ cool-down (15 minutes)

- 5-minute moderate CV exercise (see page 24)
- SMR foam rolling (see pages 44–53)
- Corrective stretching (see 'Static stretches', pages 56–65)

prone isolation abs

reps 15
sets 1–2
tempo 4-2-2
benefits increases core stabilization

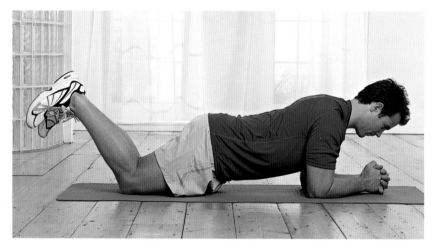

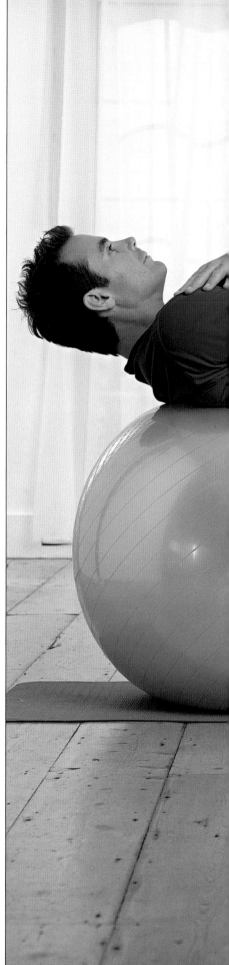

Begin by lying on your front on the floor with your feet raised and your forearms resting flat on the floor. Activate your core by drawing your navel towards your spine and squeezing your buttocks. Still resting on your forearms, lift your hips off the floor until your body forms a straight line from your head to your knees. Hold then slowly return to your starting position. Touch the floor momentarily then repeat.

common fault

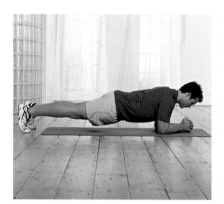

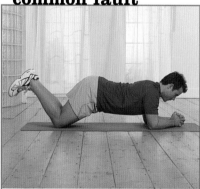

progression Increase the intensity of the exercise by lifting your entire body off the floor and supporting it on your toes instead of your knees.

Be careful not to arch your lower back. Keep your knees, hips and shoulders aligned.

ball crunch

reps 15
sets 1–2
tempo 4-2-2
benefits improves the entire abdominal musculature

1 Start by sitting on the Swiss ball then slowly roll down the ball until it is in the small of your back. Be sure you are balanced when your back is fully extended. Keep your feet pointing straight ahead, aligning them directly beneath your knees. Activate your core by drawing your navel towards your spine and squeezing your buttocks.

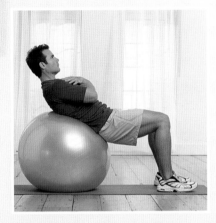

2 Contract your abdominals while flexing your hips and bringing your upper body to an upright position on the ball. Slowly lower your upper body to your starting position and repeat.

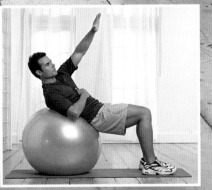

progression Rotate your upper body at the top of the movement, by stretching across your body first with one arm, then the other.

multi-direction hop

reps	6
sets	1–2
tempo	land and hold for 3 seconds
benefits	improves integrated total body stability and strength (i.e. landing mechanics)

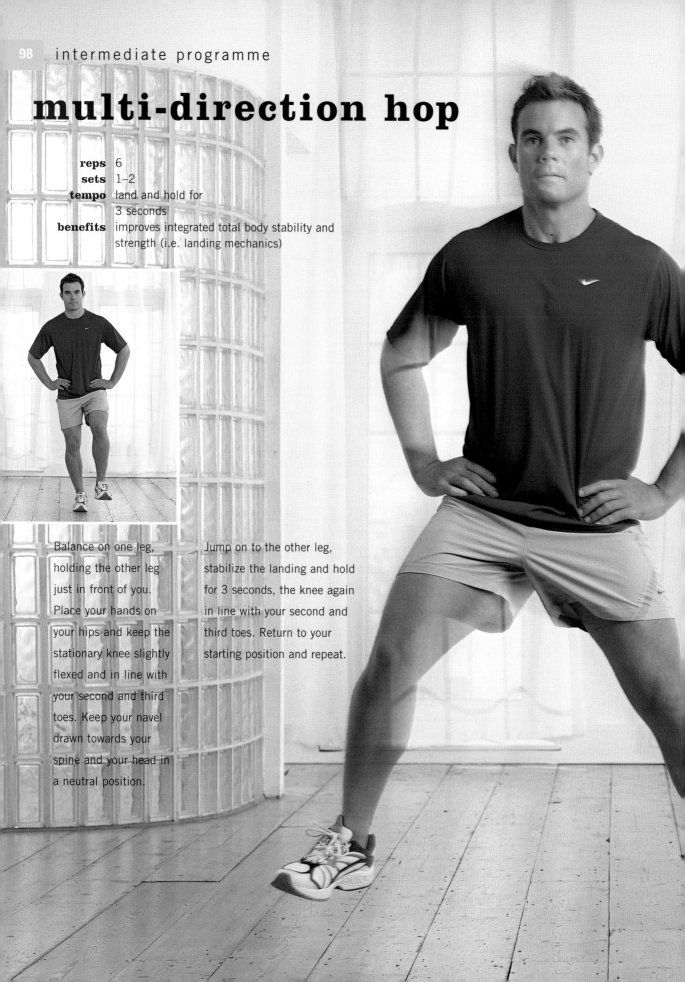

Balance on one leg, holding the other leg just in front of you. Place your hands on your hips and keep the stationary knee slightly flexed and in line with your second and third toes. Keep your navel drawn towards your spine and your head in a neutral position.

Jump on to the other leg, stabilize the landing and hold for 3 seconds, the knee again in line with your second and third toes. Return to your starting position and repeat.

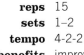

reps	15
sets	1–2
tempo	4-2-2
benefits	improves total body stability and balance, and mind-muscle connection

balance

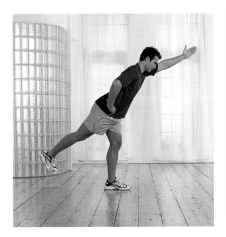

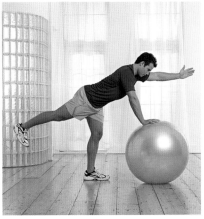

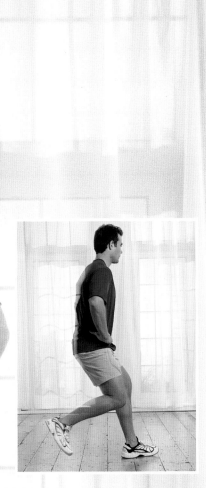

progression Utilize the same format to rotate your body and hop to a new position behind you, 45° from your starting position.

1 Balance on one leg, extending the other leg behind you. Rest a hand on the hip of the raised leg and extend the other arm out in front of you, to form a straight line from the extended hand to the extended foot. Keep your navel drawn towards your spine and your head in a neutral position. Bend forward from the hip standing extending the raised leg straight behind you, with no bend in the knee. Stabilize yourself, keeping the knee of the stationary leg over the second and third toes. Hold then return to your starting position and repeat.

progression Balance the arm formerly resting on your hip on a Swiss ball instead.

common fault

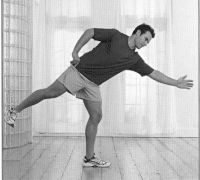

Do not bend your leg or let the extended arm come out of alignment.

squat single-leg balance

reps	12
sets	1–2
tempo	3-2-1
benefits	improves overall total body strength and balance

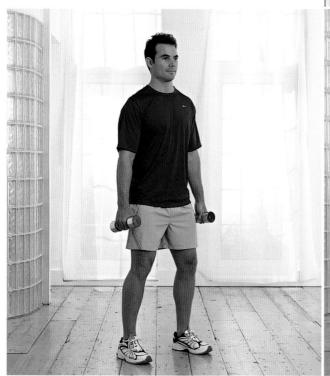

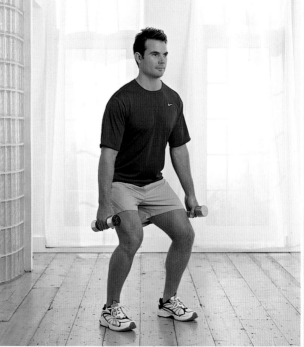

1 Stand with your legs shoulder width apart, your knees in line with your second and third toes, your shoulders down and facing back. Hold your arms down by your sides with a dumbbell in each hand. Draw your navel towards your spine.

2 Squat down in a controlled manner, bending your ankles and knees and pushing your bottom and hips behind you as though about to sit down.

3 Come back up to a standing position balanced on one leg, maintaining your entire body in a neutral position. Hold then return to your starting position and repeat the move with the other leg.

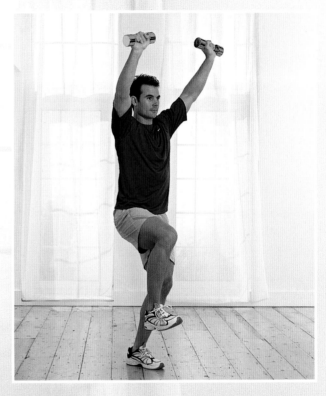

progression Hold the dumbbells above your head while balancing on one leg.

common fault

Take care not to drop your hips, knees and toes out of alignment.

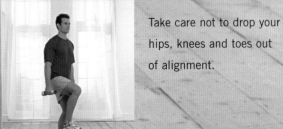

swiss ball t-row

reps 12
sets 1–2
tempo 3-2-1
benefits builds strength in the back and shoulders

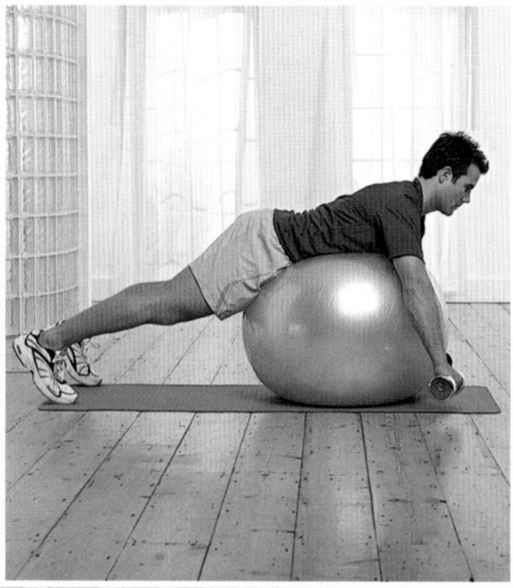

1 Lie face down over a Swiss ball with your lower abdominals and hips on the ball and your legs extended. Maintain a neutral spine position, keep your shoulders down and facing back, and your chin tucked in to ensure good alignment. Activate your core by drawing your navel towards your spine. Hold a dumbbell in each hand in front of you.

2 Bring the weights in towards your chest in a rowing action, keeping your elbows wide and knuckles facing upwards. Return to your starting position then repeat.

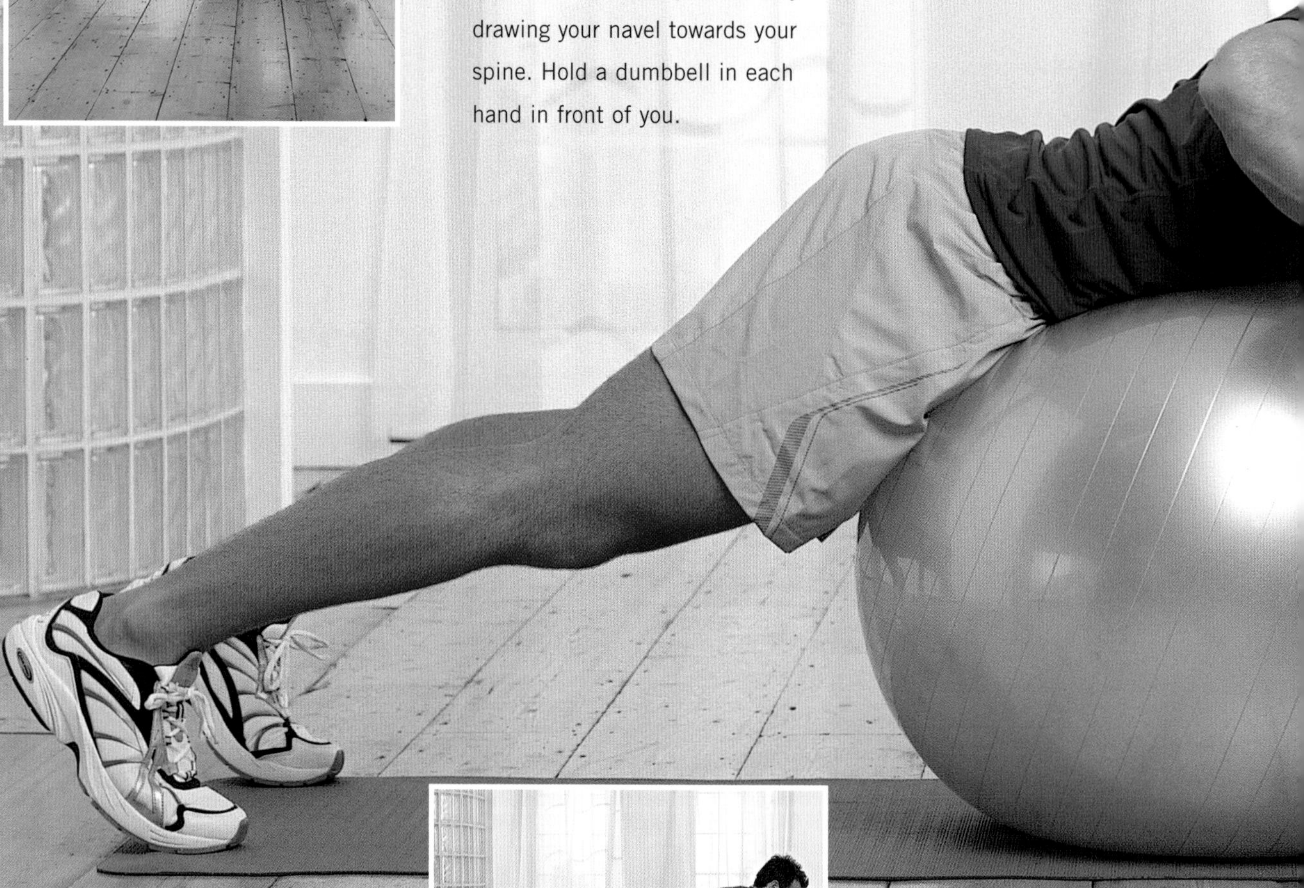

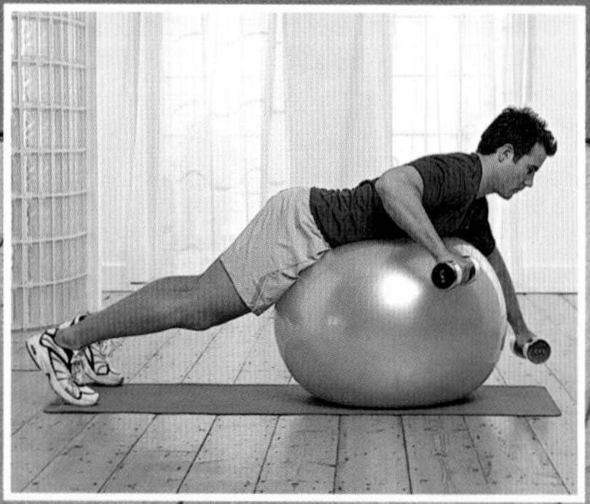

progression Bring one arm at a time in towards your chest.

swiss ball chest press

reps 12
sets 1–2
tempo 3-2-1
benefits strengthens the chest and supports the core

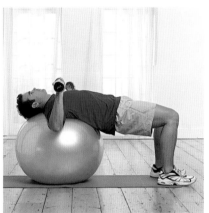

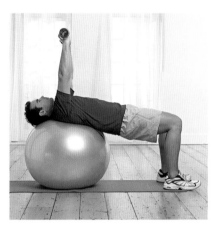

1 Holding a dumbbell in each hand, sit on a Swiss ball. Slowly roll down the ball until your head and neck are comfortably positioned on the ball and your feet are flat on the floor, pointing straight ahead and shoulder width apart. Raise your hips until they are in line with both your knees and your shoulders. Bend your arms and hold them at right-angles, pointing the dumbbells towards the ceiling. Activate your core by drawing your navel towards your spine.

2 Slowly raise the dumbbells as far as you can towards the ceiling, while maintaining a neutral spine position and stable core. Bring the dumbbells back down to your starting position and repeat the movement.

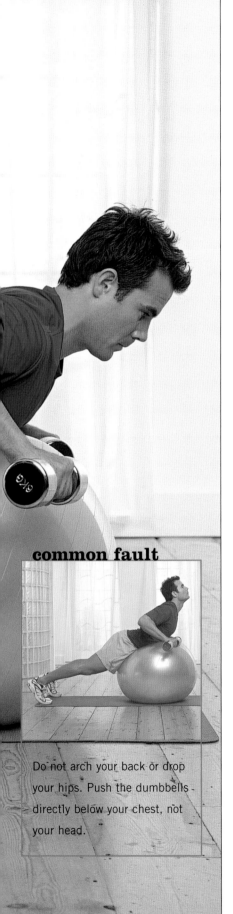

common fault

Do not arch your back or drop your hips. Push the dumbbells directly below your chest, not your head.

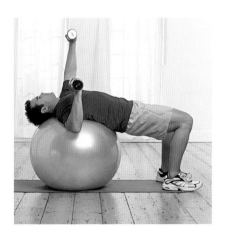

progression Raise a single arm at a time.

swiss ball military press

reps 12
sets 1–2
tempo 3-2-1
benefits builds strength in the shoulders and upper back; great exercise for strengthening the rotator cuff group of muscles (the shoulder girdle)

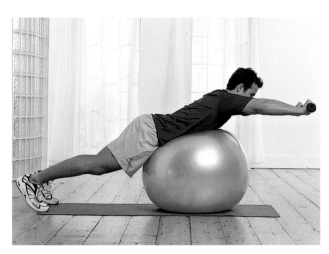

1 Lie face down over a Swiss ball with your lower abdominals and hips on the ball and your legs extended. Maintain a neutral spine position, keep your shoulders down and facing back and your chin tucked in to ensure good alignment. Activate your core by drawing your navel towards your spine. Hold a dumbbell in each hand near your shoulders.

2 Perform a military-style press by pushing the weights away straight in front of you, in line with the rest of your body. Return to your starting position then repeat.

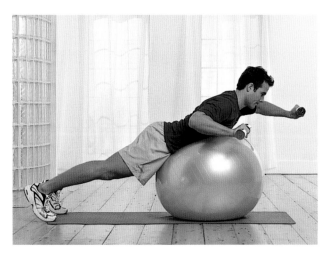

progression Extend one arm at a time away from your body.

common fault

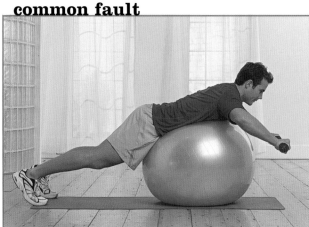

Do not arch your back, lift your head or drop the dumbbells forwards.

standing scaption

reps	12
sets	1–2
tempo	3-2-1
benefits	strengthens the rotator cuff group of muscles (the shoulder girdle)

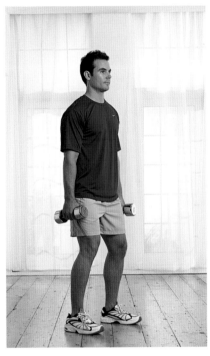 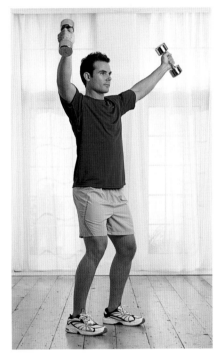 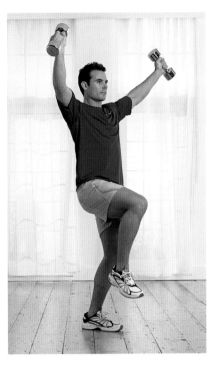

1 Stand with your legs shoulder width apart and your arms down by your sides with a lightweight dumbbell in each hand. Activate your core by drawing your navel towards your spine. Maintain a neutral spine position and ensure your shoulders are down and facing back.

2 Raising your arms from your shoulder joints, turn both arms out until your chest is open. Then return to your starting position and repeat.

progression Perform the exercise standing on just one leg.

common fault

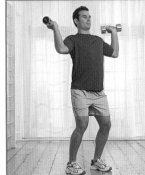

Take care not to arch your back or bend your elbows when raising your arms.

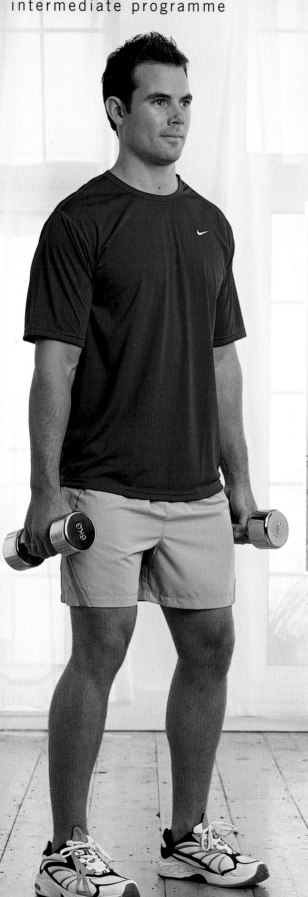

1 Stand with your legs shoulder width apart, your knees in line with your second and third toes and your arms down by your sides with a dumbbell in each hand. Draw your navel towards your spine.

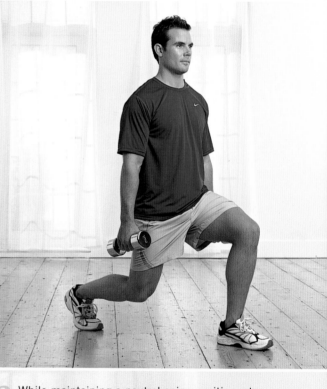

2 While maintaining a neutral spine position, step forwards and lower yourself slowly by flexing your hips, knees and ankles. Keep your torso erect and maintain the weight distribution between your heels and mid-feet. Do not allow your feet to fall inwards or shift outwards. Only descend as far as you can while maintaining your alignment throughout.

reps	12
sets	1–2
tempo	3-2-1
benefits	strengthens the legs and improves total body stability

lunge

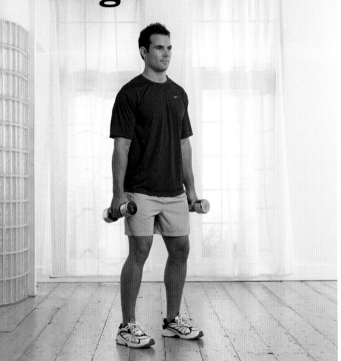

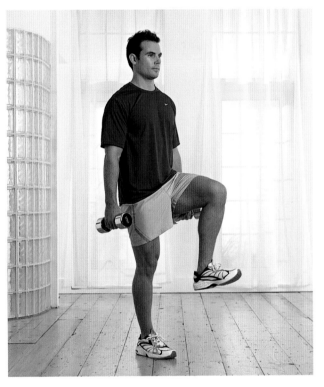

3 Return slowly to your starting position then repeat. Perform the downwards reps slowly, concentrating on the descent and the alignment of your body. Do 2 sets of 12 reps on each leg.

progression Complete each movement by returning to a single-leg balance.

common fault

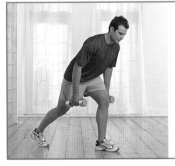

Take care not to lean forwards and position your knee over the front ankle. Don't let your feet cave in or shift out.

Challenge yourself progressively on each exercise to get the results you desire.

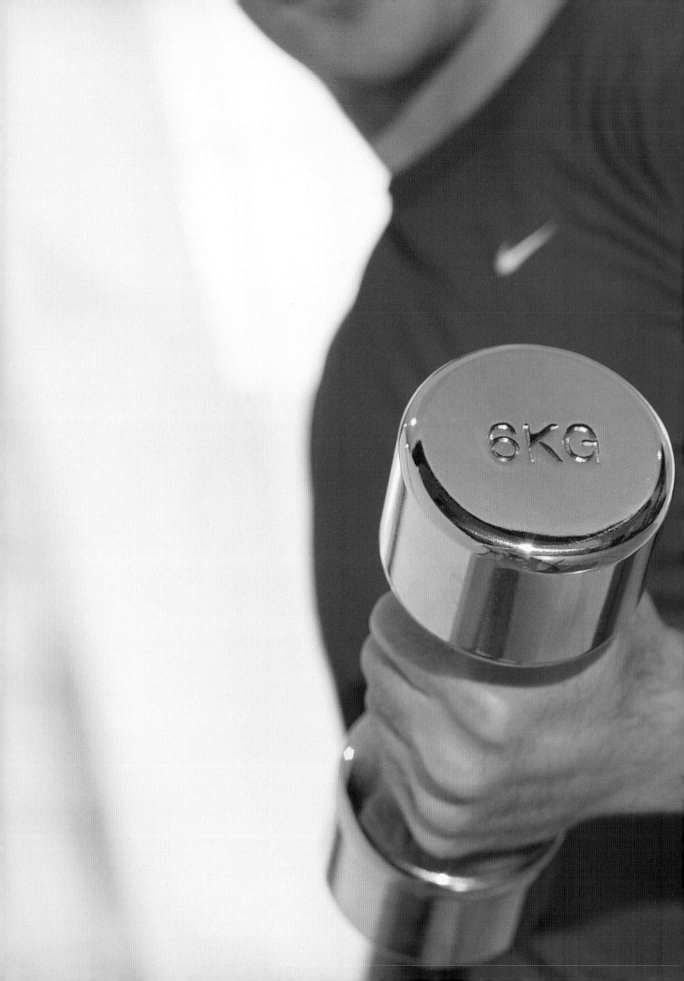

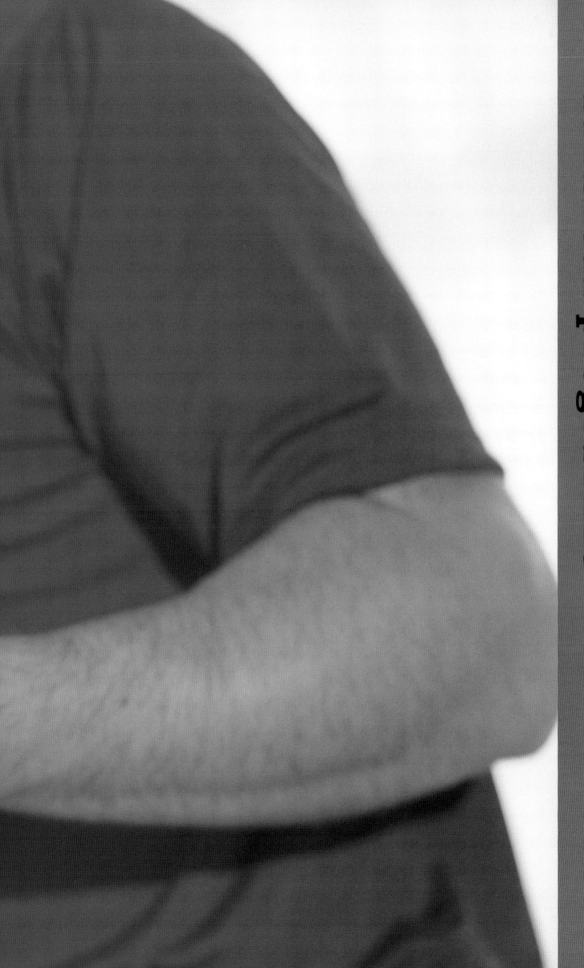

weeks 9-12
advanced programme

advanced programme

After the previous eight weeks of training you should now be prepared to launch into the final four weeks of the programme and take on a higher level of intensity with a more traditional approach to resistance and CV training. The intensive part of the programme is designed to build muscular strength and increase cardiovascular endurance, without neglecting other aspects like balance, reactive and core training. The intensive programme is broken up into two workouts (see below) – one for the upper body and the other for the lower body. Once again, the CV training can be done at the end of the body conditioning exercises or on its own on another day with a full warm-up and cool-down.

The advanced programme should take you 35–45 minutes, in addition to the warm-up and cool-down, and you should do it three times a week.

weeks 9–12 programme order

■ warm-up (15 minutes)

- SMR foam rolling (see pages 44–53)
- Corrective stretching (see 'Active stretches', pages 66–75)
- 5-minute moderate CV exercise (see page 24)

■ body conditioning exercises 1 or 2

■ upper body workout

- Supine bridge on Swiss ball (see pages 112–113)
- Prone bridge on Swiss ball (see page 114)
- Swiss ball chop (see pages 114–115)
- Lunge single-leg balance (see pages 116–117)
- Tuck jump (optional) (see pages 118–119)
- Swiss ball chest press (see pages 120–121)
- Swiss ball fly (see page 121)
- Swiss ball T-row (see page 122)
- Standing row (see pages 122–123)
- Seated dumbbell press (see page 125)
- Bicep curl (see pages 124–125)
- Dips (see page 126)

■ lower body workout

- Supine bridge on Swiss ball (see pages 112–113)
- Prone bridge on Swiss ball (see page 114)
- Swiss ball chop (see pages 114–115)
- Lunge single-leg balance (see pages 116–117)
- Tuck jump (optional) (see pages 118–119)
- Side lunge (see pages 126–127)
- Squat (see page 129)
- Lunge (see pages 128–129)
- Swiss ball leg curl (see pages 130–131)
- Calf raises (see page 130)

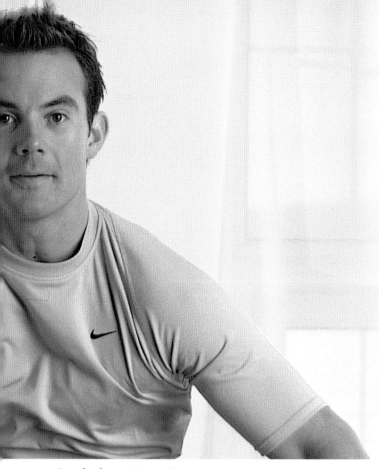

■ cv training 1 or 2

■ cv training 1

- **Intensity:** 50–65 per cent of your maximum heart rate
- **Duration:** 45 minutes
- **Frequency:** twice a week – after the body conditioning exercises, or on alternate days to the exercises

■ cv training 2

- **Intensity:** Interval training, i.e. 60 per cent of your maximum heart rate for 1 minute/85 per cent of your maximum heart rate for 1 minute, consecutively
- **Duration:** 30 minutes
- **Frequency:** twice a week – after the body conditioning exercises, or on alternate days to the exercises

■ cool-down (15 minutes)

- 5-minute moderate CV exercise (see page 24)
- SMR foam rolling (see pages 44–53)
- Corrective stretching (see 'Active stretches', pages 66–73)

supine bridge on swiss ball

reps 15
sets 2
tempo 4-2-2
benefits improves core stabilization

1 Start by sitting on the Swiss ball then gently walk your feet out and lay back on the ball. Your head and shoulders should be supported by the ball, your feet flat on the floor and pointing straight ahead, your knees and toes shoulder width apart. Activate your core by drawing your navel towards your spine and squeezing your buttocks.

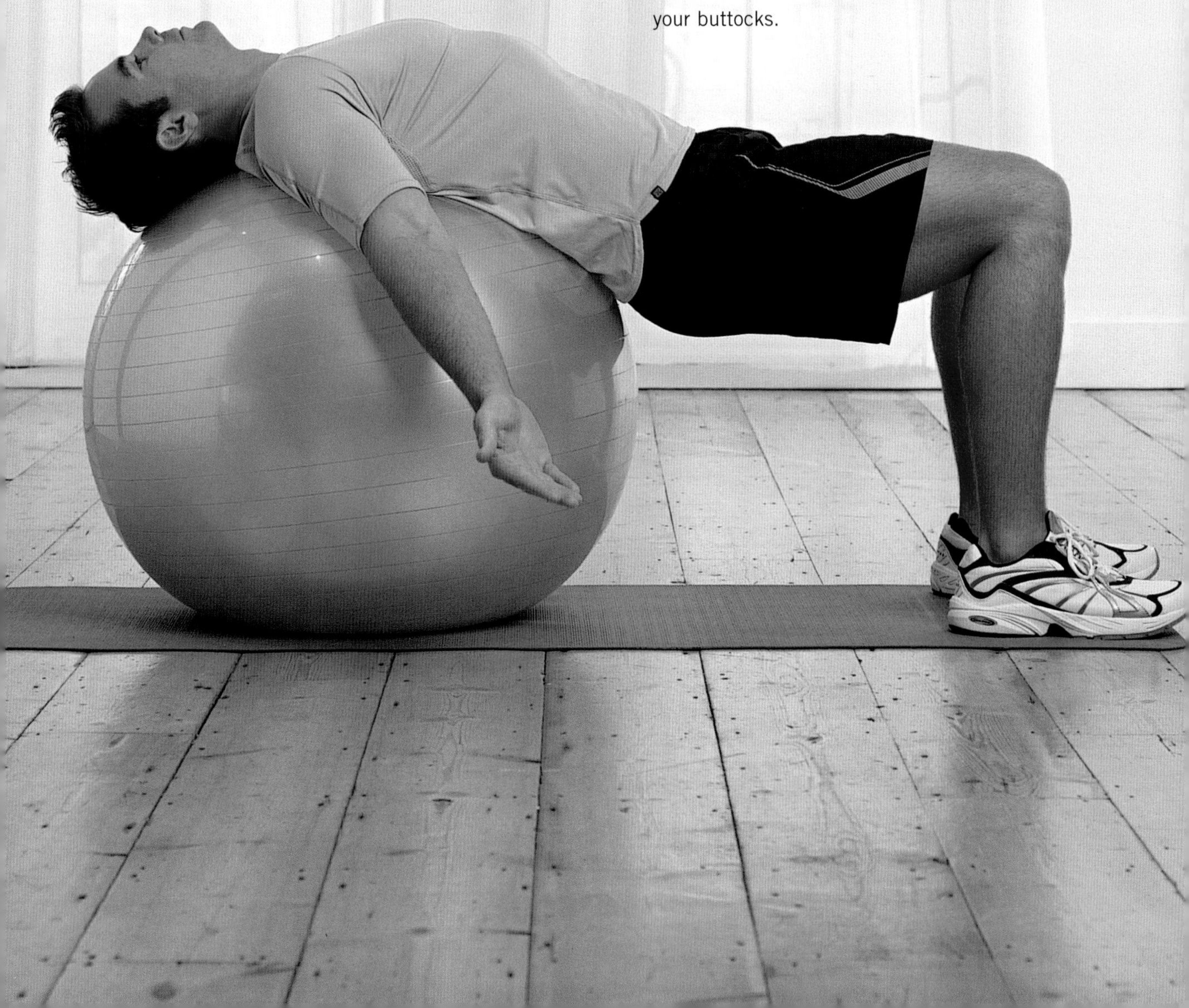

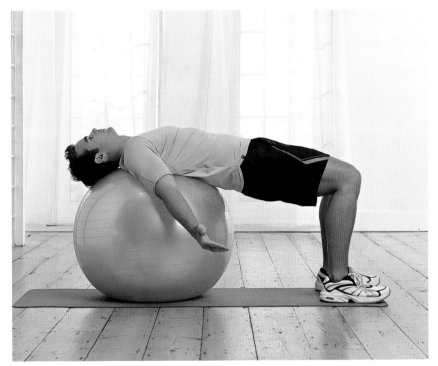

2 Lift your hips towards the ceiling to form a straight line between your knees and shoulders. Hold then slowly return to your starting position and repeat.

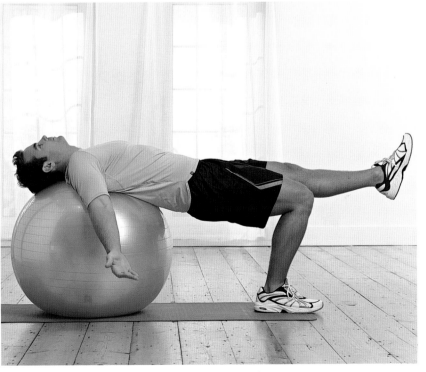

progression Increase the intensity of the exercise by balancing on one leg when you raise your hips.

common fault

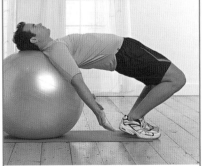

The ball should not move your knees from above your ankles.

prone bridge on swiss ball

reps 1
sets 2
tempo hold for 10–15 seconds
benefits provides stability to the core under movement

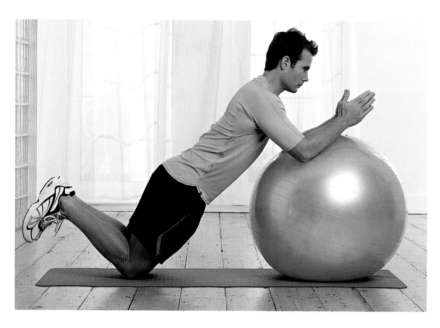

Lean forwards to rest your forearms and hands on the ball, about shoulder width apart. Position your knees on the floor slightly less than shoulder width apart and raise your feet. Activate your core by drawing your navel towards your spine and squeezing your buttocks. Ensure your shoulders are down and facing back. Still resting on your forearms, lift your hips and raise yourself up until your body forms a straight line from your head to your knees. Ensure your shoulders, hips and knees are aligned with each other. Hold the position on the ball then return to your starting position and repeat.

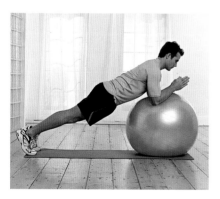

progression Increase the intensity of the exercise by lifting up your entire body and supporting it on your toes instead of your knees.

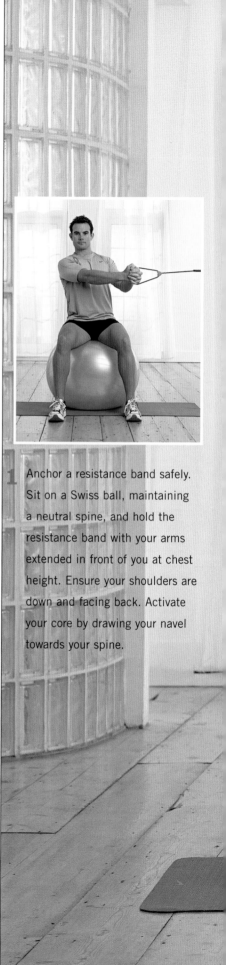

Anchor a resistance band safely. Sit on a Swiss ball, maintaining a neutral spine, and hold the resistance band with your arms extended in front of you at chest height. Ensure your shoulders are down and facing back. Activate your core by drawing your navel towards your spine.

swiss ball chop

reps	15
sets	2
tempo	4-2-2
benefits	improves core stability, posture and the whole nervous system

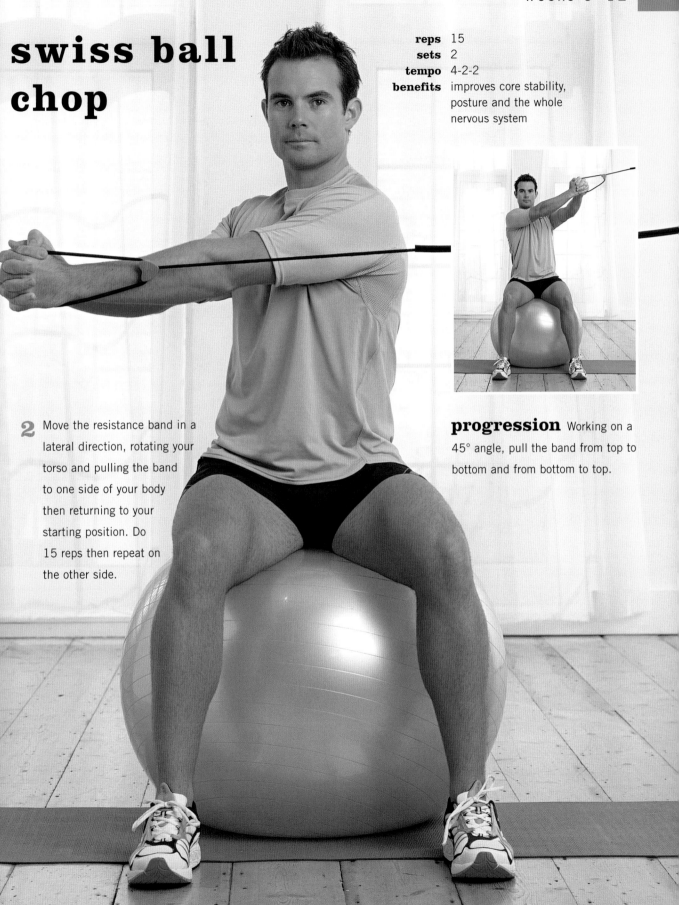

2 Move the resistance band in a lateral direction, rotating your torso and pulling the band to one side of your body then returning to your starting position. Do 15 reps then repeat on the other side.

progression Working on a 45° angle, pull the band from top to bottom and from bottom to top.

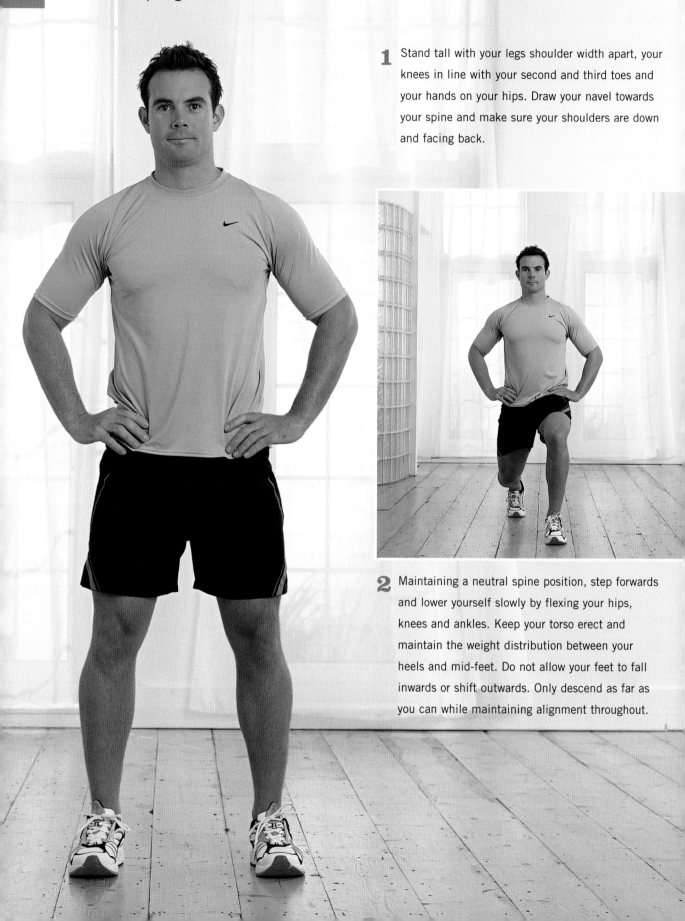

1 Stand tall with your legs shoulder width apart, your knees in line with your second and third toes and your hands on your hips. Draw your navel towards your spine and make sure your shoulders are down and facing back.

2 Maintaining a neutral spine position, step forwards and lower yourself slowly by flexing your hips, knees and ankles. Keep your torso erect and maintain the weight distribution between your heels and mid-feet. Do not allow your feet to fall inwards or shift outwards. Only descend as far as you can while maintaining alignment throughout.

reps	12
sets	2
tempo	3-2-1
benefits	improves the body's ability to balance, stabilize and decelerate

lunge single-leg balance

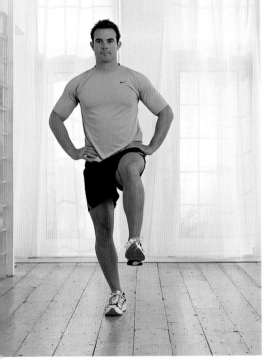

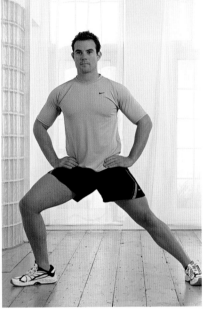

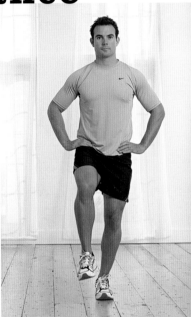

progression Working at a 45° angle to your body, lunge to each side in turn.

3 Return slowly to an upright position, balancing on your rear leg, then repeat. Perform the downward reps slowly, concentrating on the descent and the alignment of your body. Do 2 sets of 12 reps on each leg.

There is no substitute

for good form. Practise

quality not quantity.

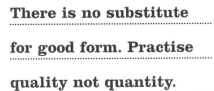

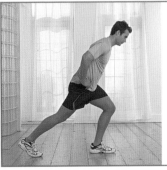

common fault

Take care not to lean forwards and position your knee too far over the ankle. Don't let your knees cave in or shift outwards.

reps	6
sets	2
tempo	land and hold for 3 seconds
benefits	improves deceleration, stabilization and neuromuscular control

tuck jump

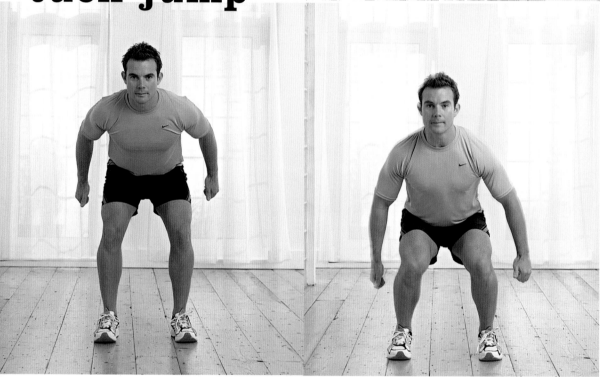

1 Stand with your legs shoulder width apart, your knees in line with your second and third toes.

2 Squat down slightly then, using your arms to help you, jump up explosively and tuck your knees into your chest at the top of the jump. Land on your toes, then your heels to return to your starting position. Repeat.

Remember to breathe

with the exercises.

Exhale with exertion.

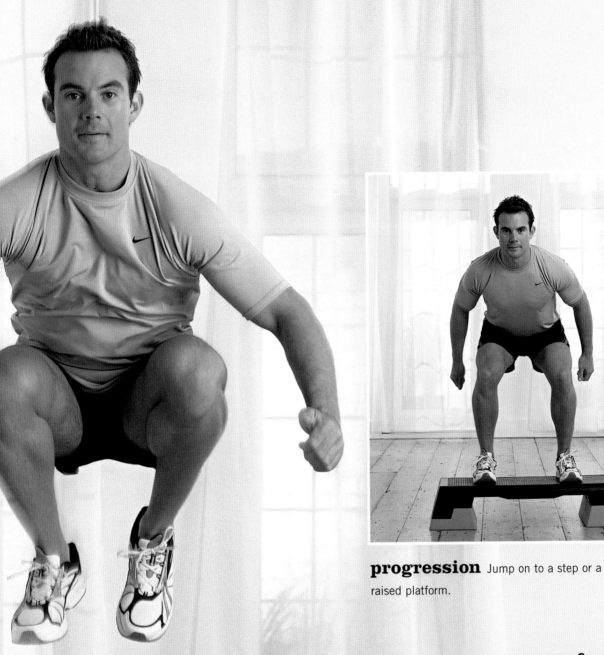

progression Jump on to a step or a raised platform.

common fault

Make sure you don't let your knees and feet cave in or shift outwards.

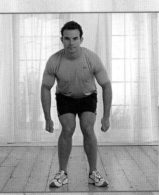

swiss ball chest press

reps 12
sets 2
tempo 3-2-1
benefits strengthens the chest and supports the core

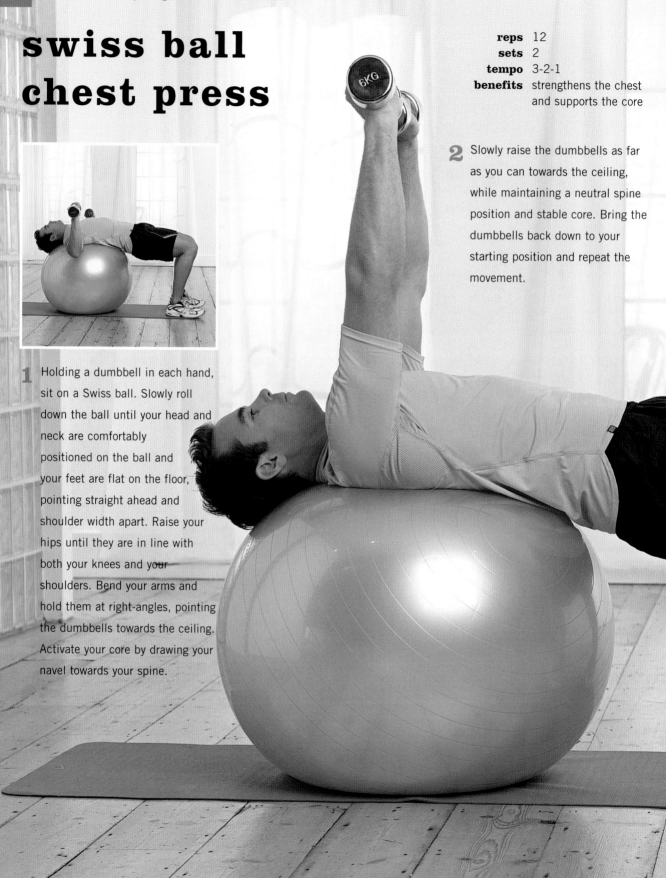

2 Slowly raise the dumbbells as far as you can towards the ceiling, while maintaining a neutral spine position and stable core. Bring the dumbbells back down to your starting position and repeat the movement.

1 Holding a dumbbell in each hand, sit on a Swiss ball. Slowly roll down the ball until your head and neck are comfortably positioned on the ball and your feet are flat on the floor, pointing straight ahead and shoulder width apart. Raise your hips until they are in line with both your knees and your shoulders. Bend your arms and hold them at right-angles, pointing the dumbbells towards the ceiling. Activate your core by drawing your navel towards your spine.

swiss ball fly

reps	12
sets	2
tempo	3-2-1
benefits	strengthens the chest and supports the core

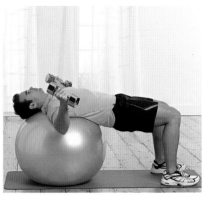

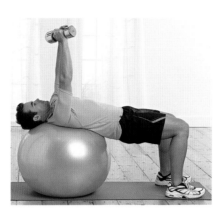

1 Lie on the ball with both feet flat on the floor, pointing straight ahead and shoulder width apart. Raise your hips until they are in line with both your knees and your shoulders. Extend your arms towards the ceiling, your palms facing inwards and activate your core by drawing your navel towards your spine.

2 Slowly allow both arms to bend slightly and lower them to your sides to about shoulder height. Return to your starting position and repeat the movement.

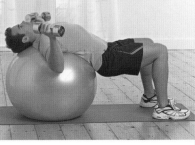

progression Raise a single arm at a time.

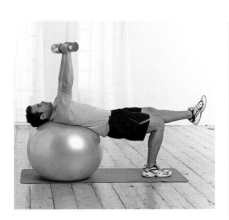

progression Perform the exercise with one of your legs raised off the floor.

common fault

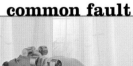

Do not arch your back, drop your hips, bring your arms down too far or bend your elbows too much.

swiss ball t-row

reps 12
sets 2
tempo 3-2-1
benefits builds strength in the back and shoulders

reps 12
sets 2
tempo 3-2-1
benefits works the whole body, strengthening the back and core

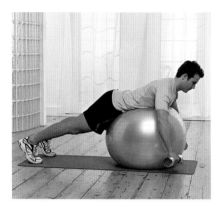

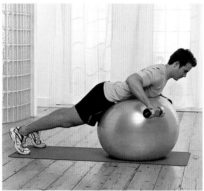

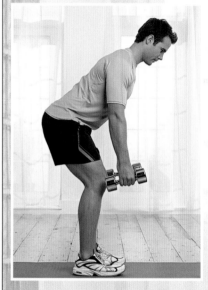

1 Lie face down over a Swiss ball with your lower abdominals and hips on the ball and your legs extended. Ensure good alignment. Activate your core by drawing your navel towards your spine. Hold a dumbbell in each hand in front of you.

2 Bring the weights in towards your chest in a rowing action, keeping your elbows wide and knuckles facing upwards. Return to your starting position then repeat.

1 Holding a dumbbell in each hand, stand with your legs shoulder width apart and your knees slightly bent. Ensure your shoulders are down and facing back. Bend forwards from the hips and maintain a neutral spine position while your arms are extended down towards the floor. Activate your core by drawing your navel towards your spine and squeezing your buttocks.

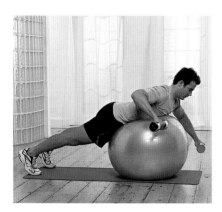

progression Bring one arm at a time in towards your chest.

common fault

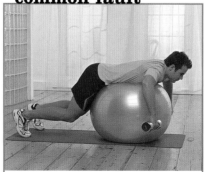

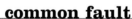

Do not arch your back or lift your head.

standing row

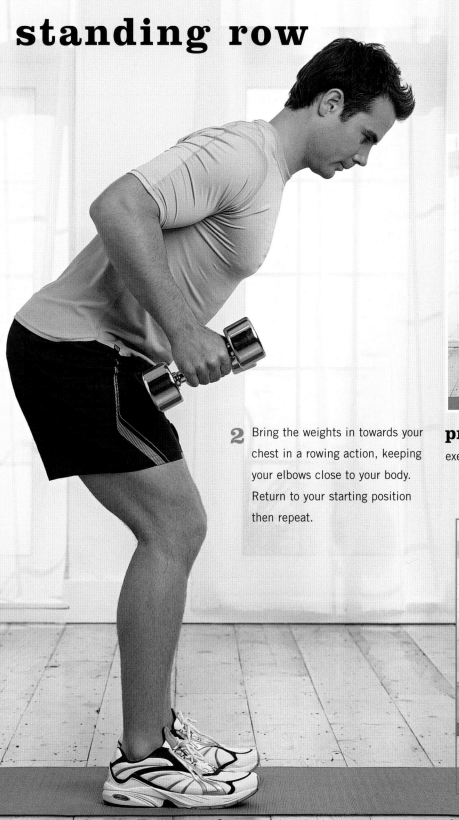

2 Bring the weights in towards your chest in a rowing action, keeping your elbows close to your body. Return to your starting position then repeat.

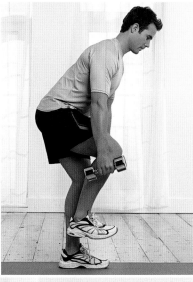

progression Perform the exercise while standing on one leg.

common fault

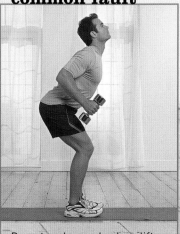

Do not arch your back or lift your head.

bicep curl

reps 12
sets 2
tempo 3-2-1
benefits improves the biceps

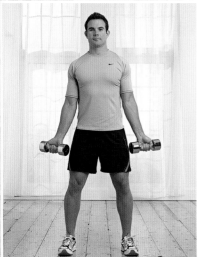

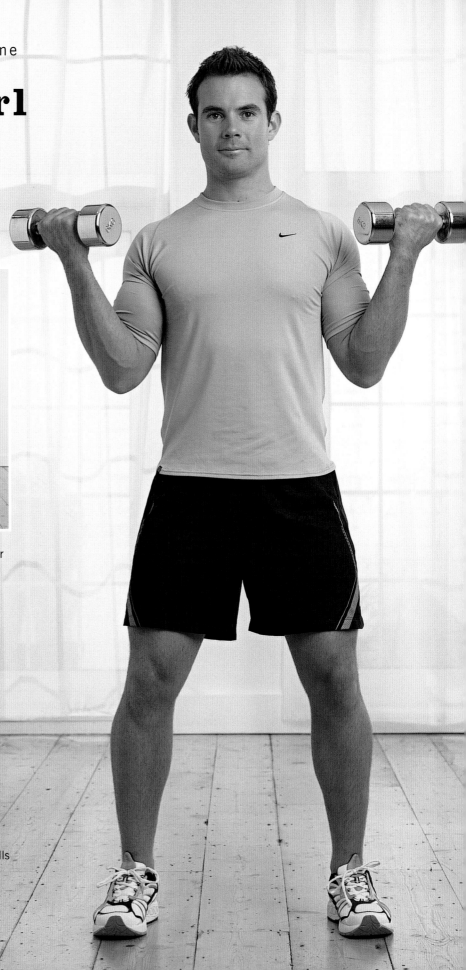

1 Stand tall with your legs shoulder width apart, your knees slightly flexed and your feet pointing straight ahead. Have your arms down by your sides with a dumbbell in each hand, palms facing forward. Ensure your shoulders are down and facing back. Draw your navel towards your spine.

2 Perform a bicep curl by keeping your upper arms still and flexing your elbows to bring the dumbbells towards your shoulders. Slowly lower the dumbbells back to your starting position then repeat.

seated dumbbell press

reps	12
sets	2
tempo	3-2-1
benefits	stabilizes and strengthens the shoulders

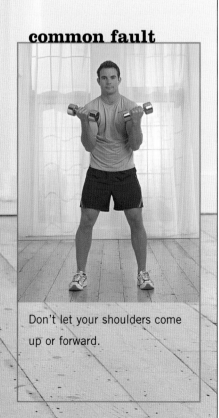

progression Perform the exercise while balancing on just one leg, then the other.

common fault

Don't let your shoulders come up or forward.

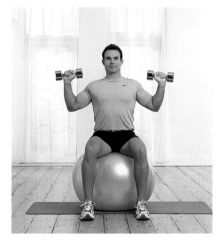

1 Sit on a Swiss ball in a neutral spine position with your feet flat on the floor. With your elbows flexed, hold a dumbbell in each hand at shoulder height. Draw your navel towards your spine.

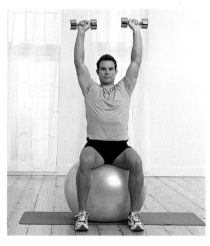

2 Push the dumbbells up above your shoulders towards the ceiling then lower them back to your starting position. Repeat.

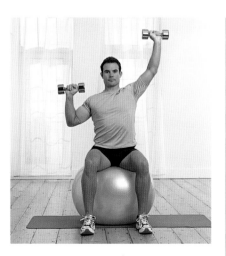

progression Raise a single arm at a time.

common fault

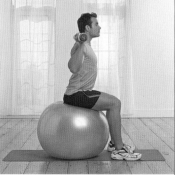

Do not arch your back or allow your head to come forward.

reps 12
sets 2
tempo 3-2-1
benefits works the triceps and chest and helps stabilize the shoulders

dips

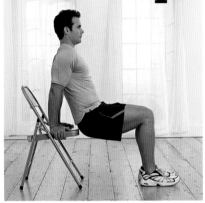

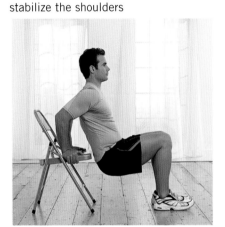

1 Grip the edge of a seat with your hands. Keep your buttocks as close to the seat as possible. Support your body weight on your hands. Keep your feet together and your knees bent. Your arms should be straight and close to your sides, and your shoulder blades down and facing back.

2 Bending your arms, slowly lower your body towards the floor until your shoulders are just above elbow height. Straighten your arms to raise yourself to your starting position, then repeat.

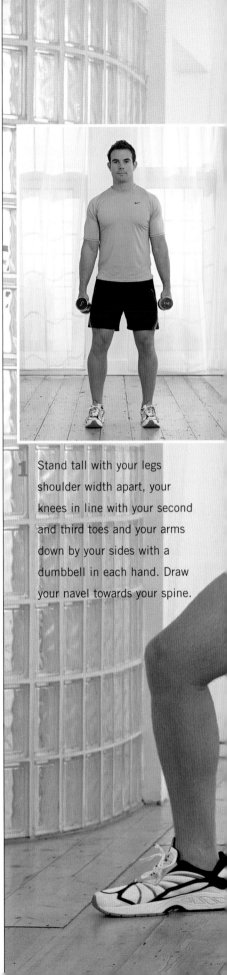

1 Stand tall with your legs shoulder width apart, your knees in line with your second and third toes and your arms down by your sides with a dumbbell in each hand. Draw your navel towards your spine.

common fault

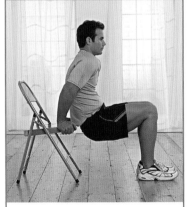

Do not let your shoulders come up and forwards as you lower and raise yourself.

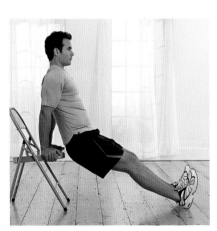

progression Make the exercise harder by moving your feet farther away from the chair.

side lunge

reps	12
sets	2
tempo	3-2-1
benefits	improves lower body control and strength in multi-directions

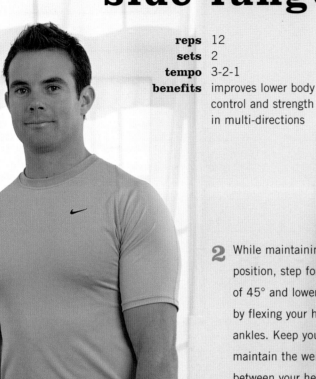

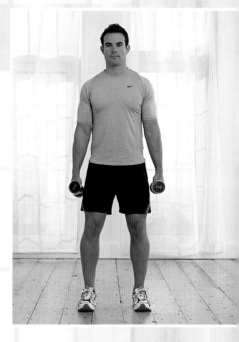

2 While maintaining a neutral spine position, step forwards at an angle of 45° and lower yourself slowly by flexing your hips, knees and ankles. Keep your torso erect and maintain the weight distribution between your heels and mid-feet. Do not allow your feet to cave in or shift outwards. Only descend as far as you can while maintaining your alignment throughout.

3 Return slowly to your starting position then repeat. Perform the downward reps slowly, concentrating on the descent and the alignment of your body. Do 2 sets of 12 reps on each leg.

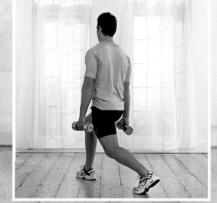

common fault

Do not allow your feet to cave in or shift outwards. Do not rotate your whole body by 45° – your pelvis should stay facing the front.

progression Rotate and step behind at a 45° angle.

reps	12
sets	2
tempo	3-2-1
benefits	strengthens the legs and improves total body stability

lunge

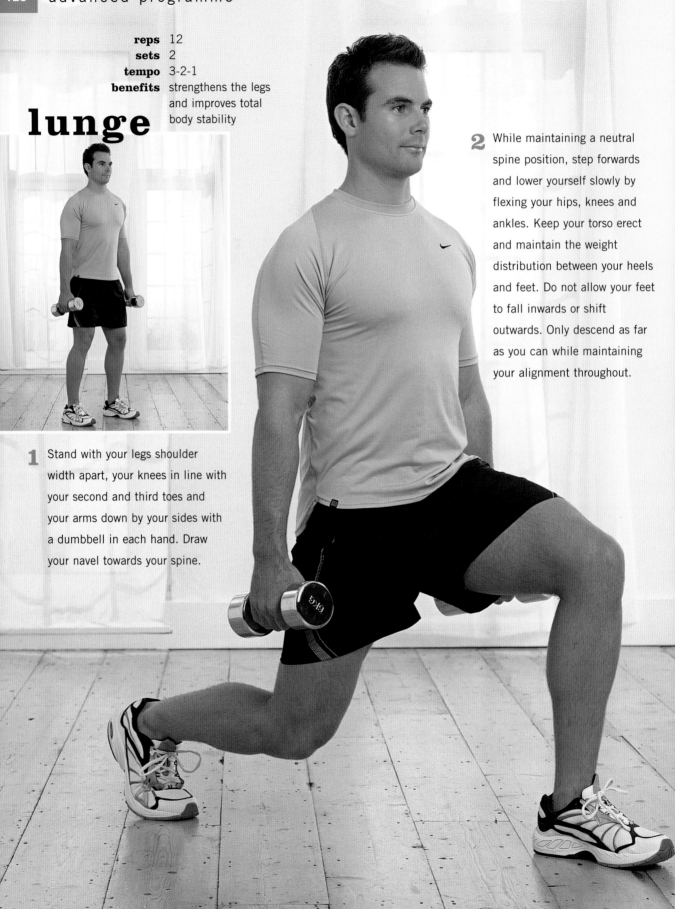

1 Stand with your legs shoulder width apart, your knees in line with your second and third toes and your arms down by your sides with a dumbbell in each hand. Draw your navel towards your spine.

2 While maintaining a neutral spine position, step forwards and lower yourself slowly by flexing your hips, knees and ankles. Keep your torso erect and maintain the weight distribution between your heels and feet. Do not allow your feet to fall inwards or shift outwards. Only descend as far as you can while maintaining your alignment throughout.

reps 12
sets 2
tempo 3-2-1
benefits improves total body stability and strength, with emphasis on the lower body

squat

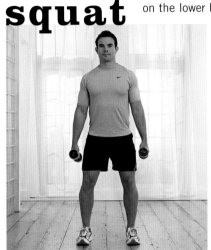

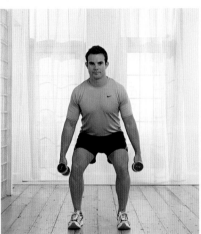

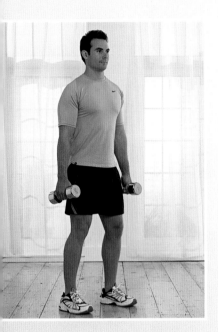

3 Return slowly to your starting position then repeat. Perform the downwards reps slowly, concentrating on the descent and the alignment of your body. Do 2 sets of 12 reps on each leg.

1 Stand with your legs shoulder width apart or wider, your knees in line with your second or third toes. Hold your arms down by your sides with a dumbbell in each hand, ensuring your shoulders are down and facing back.

2 Draw your navel towards your spine. Keeping your shoulders down and facing back, and your spine neutral, lower yourself slowly into a squat position by bending at the knees and hips, pushing your bottom and hips behind you as though about to sit down. Return to your starting position and repeat. Perform the downwards reps slowly and concentrate on the descent and the finish position. Descend as far as you can while still maintaining good control. Partial squats should progress to full squats as you improve.

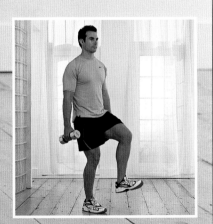

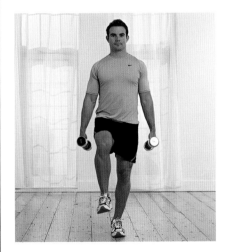

progression Complete each movement by returning to a single-leg balance.

progression Perform the exercise while standing on just one leg, then the other.

reps 12
sets 2
tempo 3-2-1
benefits works the hamstrings and core
using the glutes as a stabilizer

swiss ball leg curl

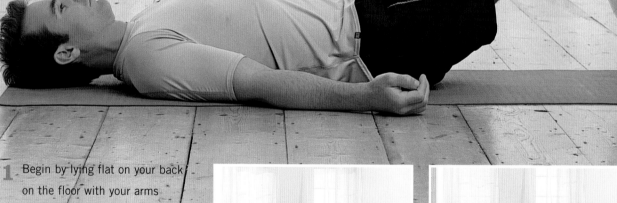

1 Begin by lying flat on your back on the floor with your arms outstretched, palms facing upwards. Place your heels on a Swiss ball with your toes pointing towards the ceiling. Activate your core by drawing your navel towards your spine and squeezing your buttocks.

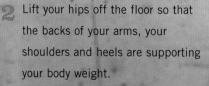

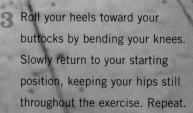

2 Lift your hips off the floor so that the backs of your arms, your shoulders and heels are supporting your body weight.

3 Roll your heels toward your buttocks by bending your knees. Slowly return to your starting position, keeping your hips still throughout the exercise. Repeat.

Reps	12
Sets	2
Tempo	3-2-1
Benefits	Improves calf strength and stability

calf raise

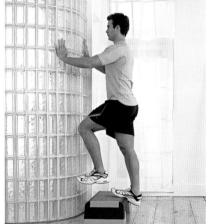

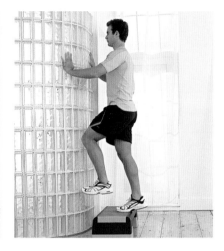

1 Begin by standing on the edge of a step – so that your heels can drop and experience a full range of motion. Your legs should be shoulder width apart and your toes gripping the floor and pointing straight ahead.

2 Keeping your whole body aligned, raise your heel and hold. Lower slowly and repeat. Do 2 sets of 12 reps on each leg.

common fault

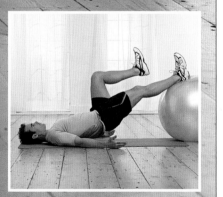

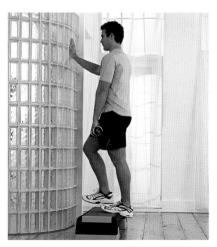

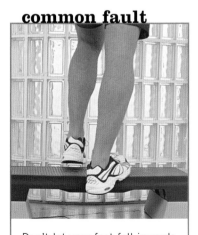

progression Increase the intensity of the exercise by raising one leg off the ball so that you perform the ball curl using just one leg.

progression Hold dumbbells to add resistance.

Don't let your feet fall inwards or shift outwards.

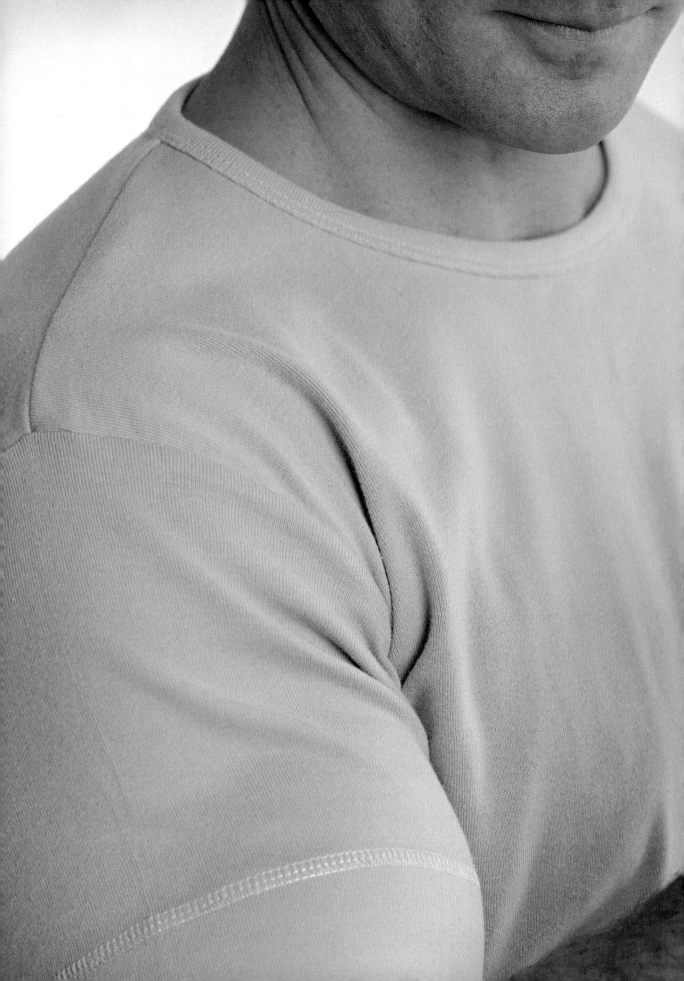

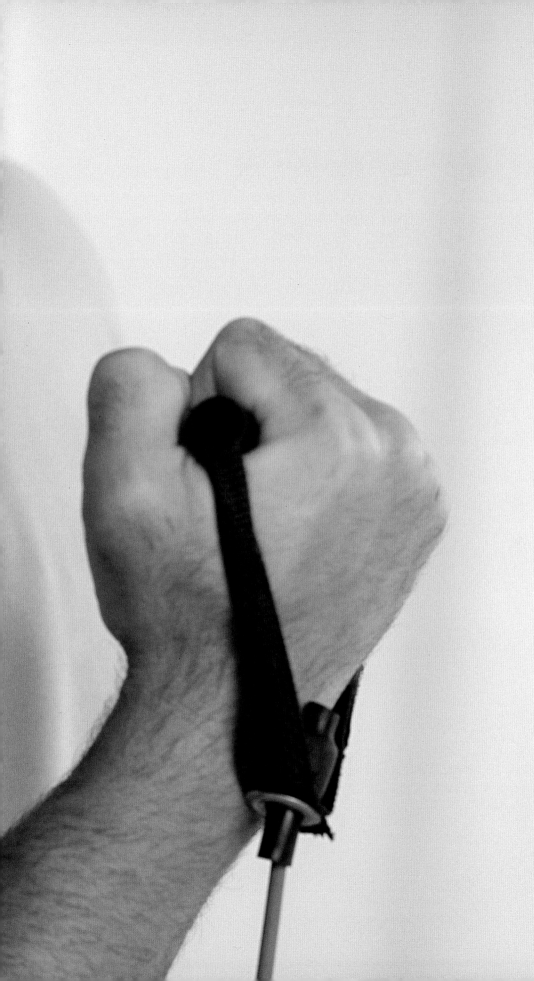

weeks 1–4
starter programme

In weeks 1–4, you should do the body conditioning exercises (see pages 44–65) two times a week. The session should take 35–45 minutes to complete, in addition to the warm-up and cool-down and any CV work. The CV training can be done twice a week, either on its own or with the body conditioning exercises. Done on its own, the training should be accompanied by a full warm-up and cool-down.

The timetable below is a recommended programme for a week, but the programme is flexible, so follow the rules above to create a programme that fits in with your lifestyle.

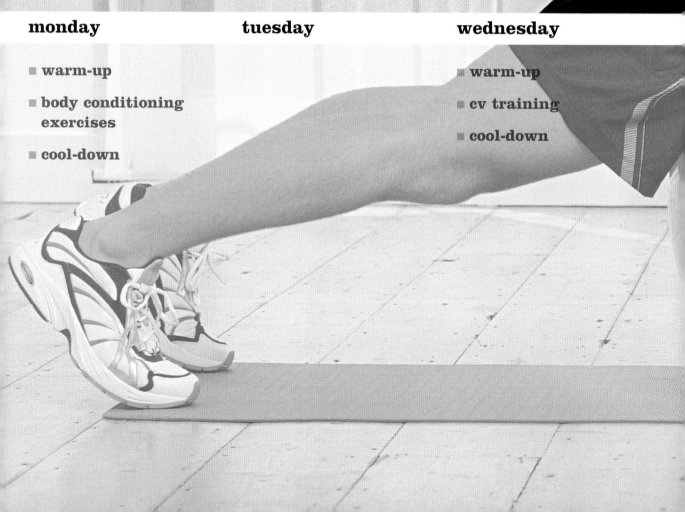

monday	tuesday	wednesday
■ warm-up		■ warm-up
■ body conditioning exercises		■ cv training
■ cool-down		■ cool-down

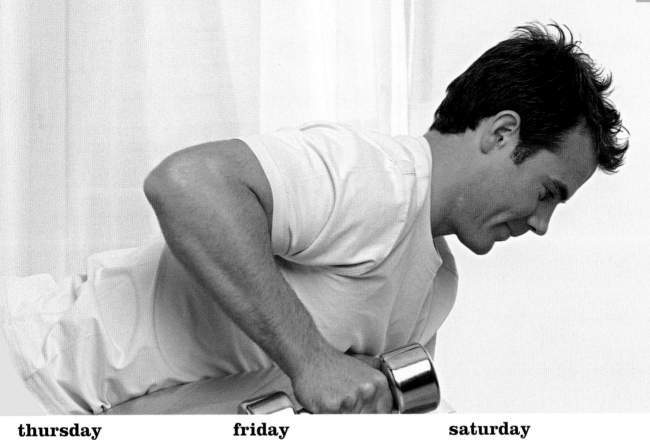

thursday	friday	saturday
	■ warm-up	■ warm-up
	■ body conditioning exercises	■ cv training
	■ cool-down	■ cool-down

weeks 5–8
intermediate programme

In weeks 5–8, you should do the body conditioning exercises (see pages 44–65) three times a week. The session should take 35–45 minutes to complete, in addition to the warm-up and cool-down and any CV work. The CV training can be done on non-body conditioning exercise days, but must be accompanied by a full warm-up and cool-down. Do CV training 1 for 45 minutes once a week and CV training 2 (interval training, which is harder work) for 30 minutes once a week, to give you a total of two CV workouts per week.

The timetable below is a recommended programme for a week, but the programme is flexible, so follow the rules above to create a programme that fits in with your lifestyle.

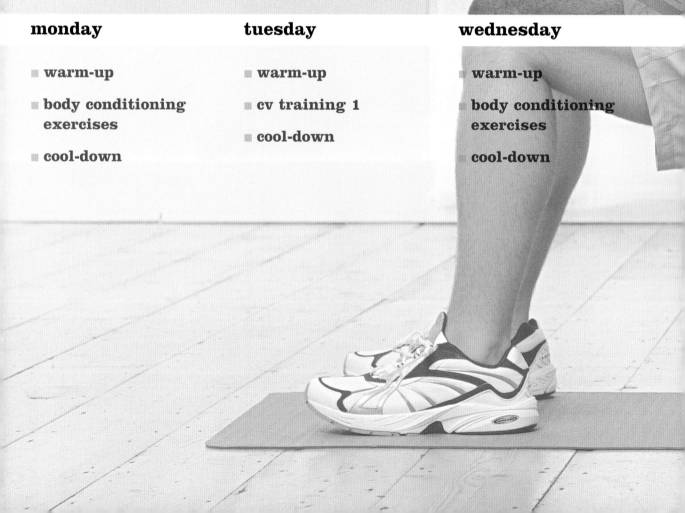

monday

- warm-up
- body conditioning exercises
- cool-down

tuesday

- warm-up
- cv training 1
- cool-down

wednesday

- warm-up
- body conditioning exercises
- cool-down

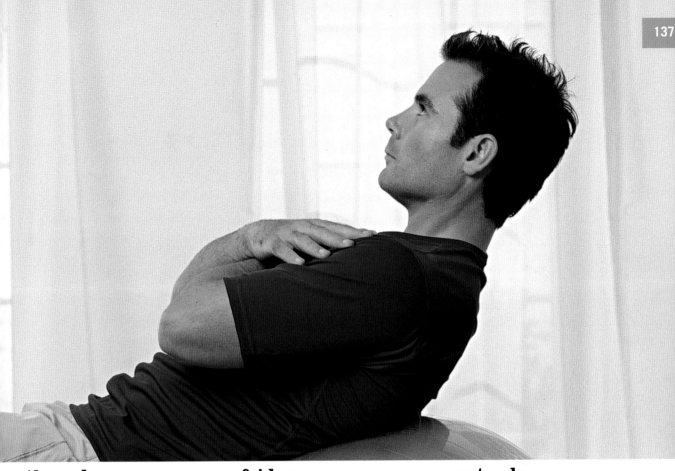

thursday	friday	saturday
	■ warm-up	■ warm-up
	■ body conditioning exercises	■ cv training 2
	■ cool-down	■ cool-down

weeks 9–12
advanced programme

In weeks 9–12, you should do the body conditioning exercises (see pages 44–53 and 66–73) three times a week. There are two different workouts – 1 is for the upper body, 2 is for the lower half – so you can vary your workouts over the four weeks (see below). Each session should take 35–45 minutes to complete, in addition to the warm-up and cool-down and any CV work. Alternatively, the CV training can be done on other days, but must be accompanied by a full warm-up and cool-down. You should do CV training 1 for 45 minutes twice a week, and CV training 2 (interval training, which is harder work) for 30 minutes twice a week. The sample timetables below will help you work out your exercise programme for the weeks.

weeks 9 and 11

monday	tuesday	wednesday
■ warm-up	■ warm-up	■ warm-up
■ body conditioning exercises 1	■ cv training 1	■ body conditioning exercises 2
■ cool-down	■ cool-down	■ cool-down

week 10 and 12

monday	tuesday	wednesday
■ warm-up	■ warm-up	■ warm-up
■ body conditioning exercises 2	■ cv training 1	■ body conditioning exercises 1
■ cool-down	■ cool-down	■ cool-down

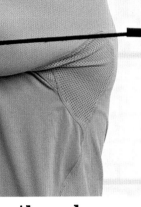

thursday

- warm-up
- cv training 2
- cool-down

friday

- warm-up
- body conditioning exercises 1
- cool-down

saturday

- warm-up
- cv training 2
- cool-down

thursday

- warm-up
- cv training 2
- cool-down

friday

- warm-up
- body conditioning exercises 2
- cool-down

saturday

- warm-up
- cv training 2
- cool-down

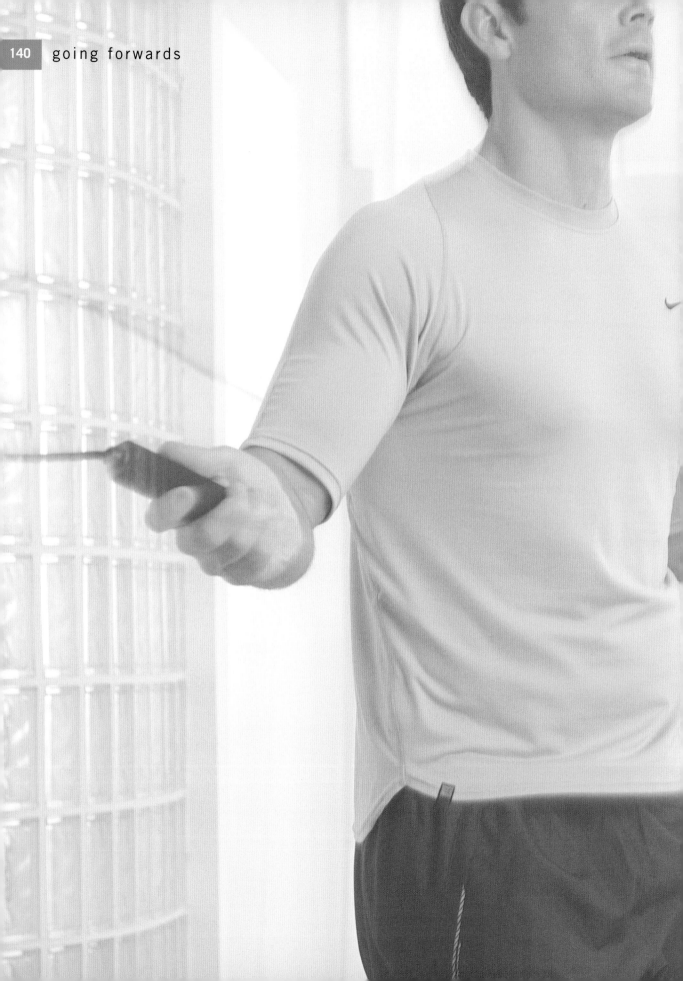

going forwards

There is always a difference between the science of health and fitness and the reality of everyday life. Quite often, the science adds up but just won't work in real-life situations because it's not really practical.

Change your behaviour

Exercise and diet are the key tools in the fight against the modern 'epidemic' of sedentary behaviour. Conditions like heart disease, diabetes and back problems are all associated with lack of exercise, so you can only be doing yourself good if you decide to make being fit and healthy your goal. The challenge is to change your behaviour and the way to do it is to do whatever works for *you*! If you are able to stick to an exercise and eating plan that is safe and realistic for your lifestyle then it will be effective. The most important factors for success are that you find your chosen programme enjoyable and practical. Only then can it help you achieve your goal.

It can also be useful to seek advice from qualified fitness professionals and registered dieticians. They can point you in the right direction, so you can be more effective with your acquired knowledge of safe exercise and healthy eating.

Your chosen programme must be realistic and address issues of:

- Safety
- Lifestyle
- Behaviour
- Habits
- Education
- Empowerment
- Exercise
- Support
- Specificity
- Nutrition

Such a programme will work because it will teach you to coach your body through a process that allows you ultimately to change your body in a manner that you can maintain. Do this correctly and, although there is a definite time investment on your part, the pay-off will be immeasurable.

Longevity and quality of life

Persistence, not perfection, will help release you from the feeling of being overwhelmed by modern living and allow you to enjoy all that life has to offer. I cannot stress enough that balance and fun is the key to being consistent with exercise. Keep your training simple and uncomplicated, fresh and new, and it will become a natural part of your daily routine!

index

acknowledgements

Author acknowledgements

First of all I would like to thank my family in London Ariane and Adriane for your love and support and to my family and loved ones in Australia for the constant encouragement. Special thank you to Mel Goldberg, the fabulous girls at Hamlyn, Mike Prior, Penny Hunking, John Hardy, Richard Boyde and (ptonthenet), N.A.S.M., Michelle Wright and Peter Goldie.

Paul Stephen Lubicz
For more information go to www.psltraining.com

Publisher acknowledgements

With special thanks to the 'Physical Company' for the kind loan of their equipment, and to Nike for their sportswear.

Physical Company
2a Desborough Industrial Park
Desborough Park Road, High Wycombe
Bucks HP12 3BG
Tel: 01494 769222
www.physicalcompany.co.uk

www.nike.com

Executive Editor **Nicola Hill**
Managing Editor **Clare Churly**
Executive Art Editor **Joanna MacGregor**
Designer **Simon Wilder**
Photographer **Mike Prior**
Senior Production Controller **Martin Croshaw**